MR. CR

I T ... A

PLEASRE MEETW G
YOU!

# 10 Minutes To Live

STAY SAFE!

# 10 Minutes To Live

## Surviving an Active Shooter Using A.L.I.V.E.®

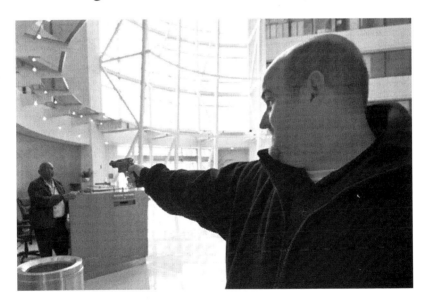

MICHAEL JULIAN, CPI, PPS, CSP
CEO/President
National Business Investigations, Inc.
and MPS Security & Protection

## NOTE

© 2018 Michael Julian, CPI, PPS, CSP
All rights reserved.

ISBN-13: 9780692992197
ISBN-10: 0692992197
Library of Congress Control Number: 2017919485
10 Minutes To Live, MURRIETA, CA

*I dedicate this book to my father, without whom I would likely never have learned so much about security and investigations or have been pointed in the direction of a career in these professions;*

*To my two children, Michael and Alexandra, without whom I would never have felt a sense of purpose higher than myself and would never have learned the true value of life;*

*And to my incredibly competent executive staff Anthony, Brenda, Dennis, Lisa, Nicole and Valerie — who because of their professionalism, skill, and dedication to running my companies so competently, I had time to write this book.*

# Contents

# Preface

For all intents and purposes, this book was complete and headed to print when, on October 1, 2017, millionaire businessman Stephen Paddock opened fire on the audience of the Route 91 Harvest Country Music Festival from the thirty-second floor of the Mandalay Bay Hotel and Casino in Las Vegas, Nevada, killing fifty-eight people and wounding over five hundred more before killing himself when police breached the room.

This was the deadliest active shooter event in modern American history and the first mass shooting from a highly elevated position since August 1, 1966, when Charles Whitman opened fire on campus from the observation deck on the 27th floor of the Clock Tower at the University of Texas at Austin. I felt it imperative that I address this event in my book and lend some thoughts on how to survive future events like these.

There is very little one can do while standing shoulder to shoulder in a crowd of twenty-two thousand people when an active shooter opens fire, but there *are* some steps you can take to increase your odds of survival, most of which should be done prior to such an event happening.

1. When entering a large venue such as the open-air location of a music festival, take note of your surroundings. Be situationally aware.
2. Ask yourself (and remember) where the entrances and exits of the perimeter of the park, amphitheater, or concert hall are located.
3. Make a mental note of the entrances and exits of the interior of the venue, including vending areas that may have a back door you can escape through.
4. Look up. As in the case of the Route 91 Harvest Festival shooter, see where someone could fire a gun with a superior vantage point.
5. Many people have never even heard a gunshot except on television. Now that footage of the Las Vegas incident has been broadcast on every news network, and the video has gone viral on all social-media sites, people know what real gunfire sounds like and can react immediately when they hear that sound rather than assuming it is fireworks or part of the show.
6. Position yourself for safety. Many people purchase the closest, most centrally located seats possible to better enjoy the show, but sitting or standing near an exit increases your ability to exit quickly. Additionally, sitting or standing near a pillar, wall, or barrier makes it possible to take cover once the origin of the gunfire is determined.

Future entertainment events like these will likely have countersnipers positioned with equally superior vantage points to respond if someone opens fire from a distance. In the meantime, it's up to you and you alone.

As of this writing, the motive for this successful, financially stable man with a seemingly good life to commit such a senseless act against humanity is unknown. This horrific loss of life should never have happened, but it was not to be the last time we'd see such a terrible incident in 2017.

## First Baptist Church, Sutherland Springs, Texas

Only five weeks later, on Sunday, November 5, another horrifying mass killing occurred, taking the lives of twenty-six people, including children, while they worshipped at the First Baptist Church in Sutherland Springs, Texas. The shooter, twenty-six-year-old Devin Kelley, a dishonorably discharged Air Force service member with a history of violence against his family members and against animals, entered the church and began randomly shooting.

It has been speculated that these murders were not religiously motivated, and that domestic violence was the catalyst, because the shooter's estranged wife and her family were regular parishioners at the church. A nearby resident opened fire on the shooter and took chase when he ran out and left in his waiting SUV. After being shot by the armed citizen, Kelley called his father during the chase to exclaim that he "did not believe he would make it." After crashing his vehicle, he shot and killed himself.

What do you do when a killer enters a church, movie theater, or other venue where everyone is lined up in a constricted area, and you can only move quickly right or left (where others are standing, sitting, or lying on the floor) or over the seats in front of or behind you? How do you protect your loved ones next to you when a madman is shooting rapidly into your area and the crowd around you? When you are staring into the eyes of a deranged person whose only goal is to kill as many people as possible in as short a time as possible, what can *you* do to survive?

If you don't have your own weapon to even the odds of survival, your next immediate actions may determine your fate. But everyone must act as a team, using the same or similar training to take down and neutralize the assailant. And where you are in relation to the killer is key to your survival, based on the actions taken by you and those around you.

When faced with this situation, you *must* stay *ALIVE*

In all of these incidents, the ALIVE response can be applied:

## Assess

When a gunman opens fire in a crowded area, people will be injured and/or killed. The total body count will depend on how quickly the intended victims react. In that split second when your brain acknowledges what is happening, you must assess the situation in an instant and decide, based on where the gunman is and your available options, what to do next—leave, take cover, or fight.

## Leave

If you are near an exit and can escape with your loved ones without drawing fire from the shooter, stay low and run as fast and as far away from the incident as possible, not stopping until you are too far away to be harmed. Call 911 as soon as it is safe to do so.

## Impede

If you are in an area of the venue where you can be hidden or can take cover behind something solid, or can even step into a side room where you can lock and/or block the door, do it immediately, leaving your belongings behind. If you can only drop to the ground, hoping the pews and/or seats between you and the gunman will stop or even just slow down the bullets, do so until the people nearest the shooter can take him down.

## Violence

Whoever is closest to the shooter must act aggressively and with the intent to kill. If a gunman is pointing the weapon to his left, the person(s) closest to him on his right must attack with all their might. Or if you are not immediately close to the shooter, but he runs out of ammunition and must reload, if you believe you can get to him before he completes his reload, do whatever it takes, with anything available, to make it impossible for the gunman to continue firing. You must commit an act of unwavering violence on the assailant with the knowledge that if you do not kill the gunman, you yourself and the people you love will be killed.

## Expose

Once the shooting has stopped, expose your position carefully. The gunman may have moved on, may have become disarmed or disabled, may be simply reloading, or may be injured but still a threat. There will be chaos—people screaming and crying and creating confusion all around you. You may expose yourself too early and still be in danger. Or law enforcement may have arrived; if you startle them, appearing to be a threat, you could be accidentally shot.

Having a security mindset prior to and a survival mindset after such an event begins is key to increasing your chances of survival. Being situationally aware—taking note of exits and barriers to use as cover and sitting or standing near them when possible—should always be considered.

These are the types of things (and more) you'll learn about in great depth in this book.

# About the Author

M ichael Julian is CEO/president of National Business Investigations, Inc. (NBI), and MPS Security & Protection. He began his industry training under his father, Ron Julian, a former law-enforcement officer and the founder of NBI. Established in 1967, NBI provides corporate, legal, insurance, and personal investigations, conducting business intelligence, theft, personal and criminal background investigations, insurance, and financial and fraud investigations.

In college, Michael majored in administration of justice and was inducted into the Phi Theta Kappa International Scholastic Order of Academic Excellence. After growing up in the family business and assisting his father in investigations during and after high school, he began working full-time for NBI in 1990, specializing in surveillance operations. Michael obtained his California Private Investigators license in 1994 and assumed leadership of the company when his father passed away suddenly in 1997.

Michael established and licensed MPS Security as a division of NBI in 2003 to provide additional protection and security services not allowed under a private investigator license. MPS Security provides uniformed physical and asset security for events, residential communities, and commercial properties; and access control, security patrols, loss prevention, fraud detection and undercover officers, and plain-clothed risk mitigation and management services for corporate, executive, and asset protection, labor-action strike security, workplace violence mitigation, hostile termination, estate security, and travel escorts.

Michael is licensed in multiple states as a private investigator and security professional and is a graduate of the Executive Protection Institute. He received the designation of Personal Protection Specialist (PPS), and he is a member of an elite international fraternity of specialized professionals known as the Nine Lives Associates. Michael's security training includes defensive and evasive driving, behavioral-threat assessment of active shooters, close protection, aviation security, and covert protection and protective and countersurveillance from Executive Security International.

In early 2015, Michael created the ALIVE (Assess, Leave, Impede, Violence, Escape) Active Shooter Survival Program, which he teaches regularly to businesses, public-utilities agencies, and medical and educational institutions throughout the United States.

Michael joined the California Association of Licensed Investigators (CALI) in 1995. He is a former district governor of CALI and served on the Legislation and Technology Committees and the Education and Training Task Force; he chaired the Bylaws Committee and held the position of vice president of administrative services for five terms before being elected president in 2012, serving for two terms. He is one of fewer than one hundred Certified Professional Investigators (CPI) and one of fewer than fifty Certified Security Professionals (CSP) in California.

Michael is the North American West Coast ambassador for the World Association of Detectives and serves on the boards of directors of the National Association for Missing and Exploited Children and the Boys & Girls Club of Southwest County in the Temecula Valley.

Michael regularly teaches courses offered by CALI and other state PI associations, as well as industry-related classes for California State University, Fullerton, and National Business Institutes on topics such as technology, personal locates, asset discovery and recovery, surveillance, and executive and asset protection.

**Praise for *10 Minutes to Live***

Congratulations, reader! The mere fact that you are reading this book means you have already taken the first and most critical step in protecting yourself and those around you. That critical first step, of course, is personal responsibility! You have made it your responsibility to do whatever is necessary to not only survive but also prevail over those who wish to inflict violence upon innocents.

Unfortunately, because of cultural changes and the untethered growth in government institutions and regulations during the last fifty years, the concept of "personal responsibility" and its true meaning have become watered down to mean "personal reliance"—a reliance on those institutions and agencies (be they municipal, state, or federal) to keep us safe. In the truest sense, we have become reliant upon institutions rather than ourselves.

Mike Julian has given you a well-researched and common-sense road map to do what is not only necessary but also mandatory for those subjected to the horror of an active shooter who wish to survive to go home and be with those they love.

Having had thirty-two years' experience in law enforcement and counterterrorism investigations at the federal level, as well as experience as a tactical-response-team commander, I can attest to the statement, "When seconds matter, the police are only minutes away!" It will be up to you!

Thomas "Mac" McCaffrey
Senior Special Agent (Ret.)

Go to any bookstore, and you'll find plenty of books about how to protect yourself and your loved ones. You'll also find plenty of nonsensical suggestions; I know because I've read a few of them myself.

If you want something more—something that's succinct in instruction and useful—you've chosen the right author.

Michael Julian has not only a vast breadth of experience about what it takes to protect yourself and your loved ones but also a unique way of connecting the dots for his readers. His writing is both sophisticated and simple, and his instinct for common sense and coherence are a breath of fresh air for the weary souls searching for real-world tactics in very serious and, too often, dangerous encounters.

As a former military member myself, I've gone through hours of emergency and weapons training, and this book is exactly what I recommend to those looking to sharpen their skills and prepare for the unthinkable.

Melissa Melendez
Member, California State Assembly

# Introduction

Columbine High School. The Century movie theater in Aurora, Colorado. Sandy Hook Elementary. Inland Regional Center in San Bernardino, California. Fort Hood Army Base. Pulse Nightclub.

When you see these locations, what's the first thing that comes to mind? If you're like most people, the answer is mass killings. Active shooters. The loss of innocent lives in shocking and horrible, senseless tragedies most of us don't and probably never will understand.

It is the goal of this book to help you, the reader, better protect yourself against losing your life in situations like these. It is to help you better prepare yourself, your employees, your coworkers, and even your families and friends so that if you *ever* find yourself in an active killer incident, you will know precisely what to do to increase your chances of survival. You will be the one who goes home that night to love, hug, and kiss your family once again.

When I give my classes on active killers and how to best survive them using the ALIVE (which stands for Assess, Leave, Impede, Violence, and Escape) Active Killer Survival Program, about 50 percent of the time, I have an attendee who says that he or she doesn't know what an active shooter/killer is. So, let's make sure you do so you know exactly what I'm talking about when I use these terms.

## Active Shooter/Killer Defined

The term "active shooter" is one we've probably heard the most in the media as many mass killings do involve some type of handgun or long gun (usually both), and many media outlets find more sensationalism in events that involve firearms. However, I often use the terms "active shooter" and "active killer" interchangeably as sometimes the weapon of choice isn't a firearm. It's a knife, explosives, or some other object capable of inflicting great bodily harm and death to many people in a short amount of time. So, what is an active shooter/killer, exactly?

The definition of an active shooter or killer is someone whose intent is to kill three or more people, usually in a confined area, and generally in places where there are lots of people to kill in as little time as possible (like movie theaters, workplaces, event centers, places of worship, and other areas where people congregate in larger numbers), and there is typically no pattern or method to their selection of victims. Essentially, the more lives lost, the more people who die during the event, the more "successful" the active killer feels.

Undoubtedly, some of what you're about to learn is going to be completely disturbing. It's shocking, really. But I want you to think about this as an opportunity to take positive, proactive action that could someday save your life or the lives of your coworkers, family, and friends. Here's your chance to learn something that could help you survive one of the most chaotic and terroristic events imaginable, so you can continue to pursue your dreams and goals.

During my in-person trainings, I show several videos of recorded attacks. They give the viewers a front-row seat to what it would be like to be there, so it's not uncommon to hear some of the attendees say, "I didn't like the videos, but I'm glad I saw them because now I know what it's really like. Now it's real to me." They feel better prepared because they're taking the class. That's how I want *you* to feel when you finish this book.

## Why You Shouldn't Go Another Day without Knowing This Material

I purposely wrote this book using as few words as I could while still creating as great an impact as possible because I want it to be a quick and effective read, without fluff that would bore you and prevent you from finishing this lesson. There are many reinforcing stories, anecdotes, quotations from other books, and other information I could have inserted to qualify the information herein, but as someone with a short attention span myself, I know how easy it is to get distracted and move on to something else, which would defeat my purpose in creating this lifesaving message.

I often relate my message directly to those who hire me to teach their employees how to survive an active shooter event, but this book is written for *everyone*. It applies to work, home, social, and spiritual locations, so, whenever I speak to anyone in this book, know that I am speaking to you.

Did you know that when an active shooter opens fire, on average, nearly a dozen innocent people are injured and killed? Look around your workplace or some of the areas you frequent where there is a moderate number of people. How would you feel if three of them lost their lives? And how would you feel, knowing that another nine or so would be lying in pain and agony if an active killer arrived right now?

Imagine too if you were one of them. What if you were the one lying on the ground shot or stabbed? What if you were the one who was senselessly attacked, even though you may have never done the perpetrator an ounce of harm?

Being prepared for events like these is the best possible tool for survival. Knowing what to expect, as well as knowing the actions you can take to keep yourself as safe as possible, is critical for you, your family, employees, coworkers, customers, and the public. It may be the difference between living to tell your own story of the event and having someone else tell it for you because you're dead.

It's no different than being prepared to respond in the event of a fire, tornado, or earthquake. We all know that these things happen, so the more we're ready for them when they do, the better our chances of survival. Well, the same is true with active killers. These events occur, and they're happening more often, so the more we know how to respond when they do, the greater the likelihood that we won't become one of the innocent victims whose picture is splashed across the evening news.

For example, if an unstable employee, ex-employee, or employee's family member entered your workplace with a weapon right this moment, would you know what to do? This is a serious question that every safety manager, human-resources supervisor, risk-management professional, employee, caretaker, and parent should be able to confidently answer yes!

No one wants to think an active killer will enter his or her workplace, but the fact is that it could happen anywhere and, perhaps most disturbingly, it seems to be happening with increased frequency. Massacres like the one that occurred at the Inland Regional Center in San Bernardino, California, where an employee left a holiday party and returned shortly after, killing fourteen and injuring seventeen others, are becoming an all-too-familiar scenario facing our workplaces and our world.

This means that people can no longer subscribe to the notion that "It will never happen here," especially given the frequency and severity of workplace attacks. In fact, that way of thinking is extremely dangerous, which is why I've dedicated an entire chapter of this book to changing that way of thinking. Too many people are injured or killed in these types of attacks because they walked into them with the mindset that "It will *never* happen to me."

## It's Time to Open Your Eyes and Train for These Events

Now is the time to adequately and effectively train yourself, your family members, coworkers, and staff how to best respond to an active shooter/killer attack, giving you all a fighting chance. Not after something has happened or during an attack, but now. Now is the time to teach *everyone* in the workplace what they need to do to best mitigate their risk of injury and death should an active killer strike.

The longer you're able to stay alive in an active killer incident, the better chance you'll have of surviving the entire event. And I'm not talking about having to fight for your life for hours either. As you'll soon learn, if you can survive the first ten minutes of the attack, then you have greatly increased the odds that you'll survive the incident.

In the pages ahead, you'll discover how to do the following:

- Identify behaviors, causes, and red flags typically associated with nonrandom workplace violence and active shooter/killer incidents before they occur.
- Develop enhanced situational awareness and a security mindset, making you a less attractive and "harder" target for an active killer.
- Train everyone around you to assure that each person knows how to safely and effectively respond to an active shooter event with a survival mindset, giving you a stronger team.
- Take what you learn and put it into action, with training scenarios for you to practice both in and out of the workplace.

## Sheep, Wolves, and Sheepdogs

Dave Grossman, a retired US Army lieutenant colonel, former professor of psychology at the US Military Academy at West Point, creator of the Killology Research Group, and incredibly pragmatic speaker, is the author of such books as *On Killing*, *On Combat*, *Assassination Generation*, *Warrior Mindset*, *Bulletproof Mind*, and *Sheepdogs*. In his writings, he tells a story of the concept of the sheep, the wolf, and sheepdog. Though many people give Col. Grossman credit for creating this concept, he explains that he learned it from a "Vietnam veteran, an old retired colonel," who said:

> Most of the people in our society are sheep. They are kind, gentle, productive creatures who can only hurt one another by accident.
>
> Then there are the wolves and the wolves feed on the sheep without mercy.
>
> Then there are sheepdogs and I'm a sheepdog. I live to protect the flock and confront the wolf.

Grossman paraphrases this ideology by stating, "If you have no capacity for violence, then you are a healthy productive citizen: a sheep. If you have a capacity for violence and no empathy for your fellow citizens, then you have defined an aggressive sociopath—a wolf. But what if you have a capacity for violence, and a deep love for your fellow citizens? Then you are a sheepdog, a warrior, someone who is walking the hero's path. Someone who can walk into the heart of darkness, into the universal human phobia, and walk out unscathed."

I want you, the reader, to keep this concept in mind as you consider what I teach you in the coming chapters. Think about this concept and imagine where the players—i.e., perpetrators, victims, *and* heroes—fit into this ideology, and where *you* fit, or should fit, when you apply "proactive reactionism," as discussed in chapter 4. Think about which one you *would* be, as a natural reaction to a violent event, and which one you *should* be. It will become all too clear how your mindset can and will dramatically affect your chances of surviving an active shooter event.

## A Passion for Your Safety

So why am I so passionate about this topic? What do I know about active killer scenarios that could possibly help you survive if you're ever in one?

I've been in investigations and security my entire life. My dad, Ron Julian, started National Business Investigations, Inc. (NBI), the parent company in Fullerton, California, in 1967, fifty years ago at the time of this writing. Then, in 2003, I founded MPS Security & Protection to offer our clients even more safety and security-related services.

As the President and CEO, I'm ultimately responsible for conducting vulnerability assessments, assisting with risk mitigation, teaching effective workplace-violence prevention, and providing executive and asset protection for my clients. I use the knowledge and skills I've learned during my training at the Executive Protection Institute in Winchester, Virginia; the Behavioral Threat Assessment and Active Shooter training offered by the Department of Homeland Security; and Covert Surveillance and Surveillance Detection from Executive Security International in Grand Junction, Colorado, where I learned about protective and countersurveillance. I pass my knowledge and skills along to others so that fewer innocent lives are shattered or lost when an active killer decides to strike.

These areas are my passion. They're my excitement. They're what I love to do. That's why, with NBI running efficiently and effectively because of an amazing administrative team, I'm moving more into the educational space, spending a majority of my time teaching people about active shooters and how to survive them. I do this by sharing the ALIVE Active Shooter Survival Program, something I've developed and trademarked to help close the gaps I've found in other training programs I've experienced, knowing that someday it will save lives.

Who knows? It may even be your life that will be saved, solely because you took the time to prepare yourself and those around you. If that's the case, then I've done my job. I've served my purpose. But understand this: whether it's my program or someone else's, the important thing is that you learn how to do something, anything, in the event you find yourself face-to-face with a person whose only goal is to take your life.

Theodore Roosevelt said, "In any moment of decision, the best thing you can do is the right thing, the next best thing is the wrong thing, and the worst thing you can do is nothing." In an active shooter situation, considering a shooter's goal of taking as many lives in as little time as possible, truly the worst thing you can do is nothing because you *will* become a statistic.

As you will read in chapters 3 and 4, I refer to the importance of your mindset, of knowing the mindset of the person intending to do you harm, and of having the correct mindset to survive when you are faced with that situation. But first, let's start with addressing the wrong mindset, which you may have already. This begins with talking about the "It won't happen to me" mindset. So, if you've ever thought that, this first chapter is dedicated to you.

## Honoring the Victims

I have described historical active shooter events throughout this book as examples of the individuals involved (both killer and victim), places active shooter events have taken place, and how the various parties reacted to those situations. But I have cited only a handful of the events that have taken place since this type of horrific event has become a common occurrence in our society. I use these examples to honor the victims of these events with the hope that the readers of this book will understand more vividly what an active shooter event is, how it comes about, and the heartbreaking aftermath of this unconscionable and senseless violence.

Though I have a tremendous distaste for perpetuating the memory of these ruthless killers by stating their names in my book, it was necessary to tell the stories of these atrocities. However, I have not included any photographs of the killers because I do not want them to be remembered as anything more than a name; I want to take from them the power they intended to maintain after their demise. My hope is that the memory of the victims and of their loved ones who were left to live with a hole in their hearts that can never be filled will live on forever. My intense desire to do anything possible to prevent the undeserving loss of life and perpetual agony of those who may lose someone they love in the future has been the driving factor in completing this book. I know I cannot stop bad things from happening, but I pray that someday, when someone who has taken my class is faced with a life-or-death situation, my teachings will give them the knowledge and confidence to prevail over that evil.

# One

## "It Won't Happen to Me"

Turn on the news after an active-shooting incident, and one of the first things you'll likely see is a reporter interviewing someone who was at the scene, possibly even one of the victims. Inevitably, at some point during the conversation, the interviewee almost always says, "I knew things like this happened, but I *never* thought it'd happen to me." Why are we so blind to the fact that this type of event not only *can* happen to everyday citizens, to the good people in this world, but it *does*?

Dr. Richard Osbaldiston, PhD, associate professor at Eastern Kentucky University, calls this way of thinking the *optimism bias*. Specifically, he defines it as holding "the belief that each of us is more likely to experience good outcomes and less likely to experience bad outcomes," causing us to "disregard the reality of an overall situation because we think we are excluded from the potential negative effects.[1]"

Put simply, believing that it won't happen to you involves having a false belief that you're somehow immune to the bad things that happen in this world. Not only is this way of thinking wrong, it's extremely dangerous.

## The Danger Associated with This Belief

Do you think that the people who went to see a movie at the Century theater in Aurora, Colorado, on July 20, 2012, ever thought they'd find themselves face-to-face with a gunman by the name of James Holmes? Or what about the holiday shoppers who went to Clackamas Town Center in Portland, Oregon, on December 11, 2012, intent on buying Christmas gifts for their loved ones, only to endure "22 Minutes of Chaos and Terror as a Gunman Meanders through the Mall"?[2]

While optimism bias is common, Dr. Osbaldiston points out that this way of thinking prevents people from heeding warnings associated with known risks, making it a dangerous way to live because you don't see the threat until it's right in front of you and may be too late to avoid. It's like being told that carrying excess body weight elevates your risk of diabetes, heart disease, and a host of other potentially life-threatening conditions but disregarding this information and being surprised when you get a diagnosis.

Several research studies have been conducted on optimism bias and have found that it is relatively widespread. One such study was published by *Health Psychology* and involved four different pieces of research performed on college students. Each one set out to ascertain the students' thoughts and perceptions regarding risk, and, after reviewing the results, the researcher concluded that, overall, the university-level participants' views "were overly optimistic" and failed to acknowledge the real risks they faced.[3]

In the case of active shooter incidents specifically, those who enter these types of situations with their blinders on, completely unprepared and disbelieving of the possibility that a person with a weapon could present immediate harm, have just moments to respond and to respond appropriately. So, if they're caught off guard by the prospect of even *being* in this circumstance, they waste valuable seconds trying to come to terms with what's evolving around them. Not to mention that the worst time to formulate a plan is when you're in the middle of a crisis and are unable to think clearly and rationally.

## Active Shooter Incidents Can (and Do) Happen All the Time, Everywhere

To change this mentality and get rid of the "It won't happen to me" belief that is so dangerous to hold, it's important to acknowledge the fact that active killer scenarios happen all the time. This begins with educating yourself about how often these incidents occur.

According to the Federal Bureau of Investigation (FBI), there were 213 active shooter incidents between January 1, 2000, and September 8, 2016.[4] Do the math, and you realize that that's roughly one person shooting and killing (or, at the very least, attempting to kill) innocent bystanders every twenty-seven to twenty-eight days.

In fact, if you look at the FBI's data about active shooter incidents occurring between 2000 and 2013, you'll notice a disturbing upward trend. During the first seven years of this time frame, an average of 6.4 incidents occurred annually. This number almost tripled during the last seven years, with roughly 16.4 incidents per year by the time frame's end.

Realistically, the true number of active shooter cases is likely much higher. Google alerts are e-mailed to me anytime this type of incident occurs and I usually receive notifications four to five times per month. However, because some incidents don't always fit neatly into the active shooter definition, they're not counted as such, which means they happen much more frequently than they appear in the news.

Take the shooting on April 10, 2017, at San Bernardino Elementary School, for instance. Cedric Anderson went to the school that day intent on killing his estranged wife, yet he also shot two students while he was there.[5] Was he an active shooter? Yes. But not all agencies would classify this as an active shooter incident, excluding it from their data and failing to capture just how often these types of incidents occur.

Look more in depth at the individual incidents, and you also quickly learn that these deadly scenarios can happen anywhere and everywhere. Case in point: here's a breakdown of the locations for the 213 identified active shooter cases in the FBI's sixteen-year time frame:

- 92% occurred in places of commerce such as retail stores, restaurants, and other businesses.
- 48% occurred in educational establishments ranging from elementary schools to universities.
- 26% occurred in open spaces or areas along interstates, at carnivals, and so on.
- 23% occurred in governmental facilities like courthouses, military bases, and police offices.
- 10% occurred at individual residences.
- 8% occurred in houses of worship such as churches and synagogues.
- 6% occurred at health-care facilities like hospitals and clinics.

Go over this list, and you quickly realize that a large majority of active shooter incidents (67 percent) take place at businesses and schools. For those occurring at businesses, while a disgruntled employee would seem more likely the cause, the reality is that three out of every four shooters are *not* an employee or former employee of that establishment, potentially making it more difficult to anticipate trouble and see it coming.

Active shooters don't necessarily stay in one location either. In more than 15 percent of the cases, the shooter spreads terror and chaos to multiple locations. Sadly, these types of "wandering active killings" will likely increase over time.

So, are there any locations that don't fit into at least one of these categories? No, which is why it's so important to realize that there's no place you can go and be 100 percent safe from an active shooter. Even police departments—a building that should be the safest place there is—aren't immune to active shooters, as evidenced by the shooting at the McKinney Public Safety building in which a gunman sent more than a hundred rounds directly toward the headquarters.[6] Even a military office is vulnerable, such as when, on July 16, 2015, Muhammad Youssuf Abdulazeez opened fire on two military installations in Chattanooga, Tennessee. He first committed a drive-by shooting at a recruiting center, then traveled to a US Navy Reserve center and continued firing, where he was killed by police in a gunfight. Four Marines died on the spot. A US Navy sailor, a marine recruiter, and a police officer were wounded. The sailor died from his injuries two days later.[7]

If you're stuck on the numbers, certain that they're wrong because you don't remember hearing about these mass killings, then you're not alone. Sure, some of these active shooter cases are well-known. Take the Virginia Tech shooting on April 16, 2007, for example. In this case, Seung Hui Cho went to the school, located in Blacksburg, Virginia, with two handguns, chained the doors shut, and started shooting, eventually killing thirty-two people and wounding seventeen more. That case was all over the news for weeks, months even.

The shooting at the Cinemark Century 16 in Aurora, Colorado, on July 20, 2012, was well publicized as well. Images of James Eagan Holmes were continuously flashed across television screens, declaring that this mass murderer with distinctive red hair went to this movie theater with multiple firearms, killing twelve and wounding fifty-eight by the time he was done. Experts probed into his personal history with great fervor, looking for every possible sign that should've alerted the people in Holmes's life that he was capable of this type of mass casualty and talking about it endlessly on air.

## Not All Cases Make National News

Most active shooter incidents aren't as well remembered because they either don't quite make it to the national news or, if they do, they aren't covered long enough to make a big impact. One example is the September 22, 2010, active shooter incident that occurred at AmeriCold Logistics in Crete, Nebraska. Just before 10:00 a.m., Akouch Kashoual entered the workplace and started firing at his co-workers, wounding three. Luckily, all victims survived, but this incident could easily have gone the other way, especially if Kashoual hadn't decided to take his own life before law enforcement could arrive on the scene (a circumstance that is common, by the way, for reasons we'll go into later).

A more recent example occurred on May 29, 2016, beginning in an auto-detail shop before the shooter, Dionisio Garza III, took his assault rifle into a nearby residential area. By the time this incident was over, one innocent person had died and six more had sustained wounds (two of whom were law-enforcement personnel).

Again, no place is immune from an active shooter incident. There's no time of day that is exempt from these killings either. Some of these incidences have happened at 2:00 a.m. (like the June 12, 2016, shooting at the Pulse Nightclub), and some have occurred in the middle of the afternoon (such as the June 5, 2014, shooting at Seattle Pacific University).

## This Way of Thinking Is Negligent

The point of providing these statistics isn't necessarily to scare you (although it should); it's to get you to see that having an "It won't happen to me" mentality is not only foolish but also negligent—dangerously negligent.

You owe it to yourself and to your family, friends, coworkers, and everyone else around you to understand and acknowledge the dangers that exist in this world. To pretend they don't exist puts everyone—you and them both—in harm's way.

To keep your eyes closed to this reality is like closing your eyes to the fact that children are curious by nature and can easily find themselves in the bathroom cabinet, taking one of the many medications that are there. Leave childproof locks off the doors, and you're inviting trouble; and if you do find yourself in a predicament where your child ingests one of these harmful substances, you may be delayed in providing an efficient, life-saving response simply because you never considered this scenario a possibility.

Don't put yourself, your employees, your family, or your friends in this situation with active shooters because you're too scared to admit that you may someday find yourself in a scenario that involves a person actively shooting at you or those around you. Instead, at least admit that it's a possibility, and then do the one thing you can do today to increase your chances of survival, as well as the chances of those around you: make a response plan.

When making this plan (and regularly and consistently training with the plan you've created), keep in mind that it's your response during the first ten minutes of the active killer incident that matters most.

# Two

## Why the First Ten Minutes Matter Most

As mentioned previously, in 2014, the FBI conducted a study on the 160 documented active shooter incidents that occurred between the years of 2000 and 2013.[8] One of the primary purposes of this research was to learn more about these types of situations, so government officials could be more proactive in preventing them from occurring in the future. Or, as Mr. Han (played by Jackie Chan) said in the 2010 version of *The Karate Kid*, "The best fights are the ones we avoid."

But the FBI had a secondary goal as well. It also wanted to create a more effective and faster law-enforcement response should an active shooter present him- or herself at one of our nation's schools, retail businesses, event gatherings, or any other location that could easily result in mass casualties. Too many people were dying in the time it was taking police to arrive on scene and take control of the situation.

Therefore, part of this study involved calculating the amount of time that elapsed from the time the shooter began inflicting violence on innocent bystanders until the threat (the shooter) was neutralized. The results?

Out of the 160 active-shooter situations that occurred during this thirteen-year time frame, the duration of the incidents could only be determined in 63 of the scenarios. However, of these 63, the incident had come to an end in five minutes or less more than two-thirds, or 69.8 percent, of the time.

As if this weren't bad enough because five minutes is hardly enough time to formulate a response, let alone enact it, some incidents didn't even last that long. In fact, in 36.5 percent of the cases in which duration could be ascertained, the incident was over within a mere two minutes, or about the same amount of time it took you to read the opening paragraphs in this chapter.

# 10 Minutes to Live

Some of the active shooter incidents that have resulted in higher numbers of mass casualties have still reportedly ended within ten minutes. Here are a few of the most well-known events that have occurred in recent history that meet this criterion:

- *Virginia Tech shooting, April 16, 2007*
  This shooting first began at 7:15 a.m., with the second attack occurring at 9:40. Approximately ten minutes later, the gunman committed suicide, but not before killing thirty-two students and teachers and wounding seventeen others.[9]
- *Fort Hood shooting, November 5, 2009*
  From beginning to end, this shooting also lasted ten minutes. In that time, twelve service members and one Department of Defense employee lost their lives.[10]

- *Sandy Hook Elementary School shooting, December 14, 2012*
  The first shot was fired through the plate-glass window of this
  Newtown, Connecticut, school just after 9:30 a.m. Between
  that time and 9:40 a.m., which is when the gunman turned
  his firearm on himself, thirty first graders and six school staff
  members sustained life-ending injuries[11].

In all three of these cases, the active shooter incident lasted only ten
minutes. While we all know how long ten minutes is, realization
doesn't often set in as to exactly how fast this amount of time goes by
until you start thinking about the things you do that take approximately ten minutes' time.


## What Can You Do in Ten Minutes?

If you're an average person, ten minutes is about how long it takes to
fold a load of laundry, scrub the toilets, or vacuum a room in your
home. Ten minutes is also roughly how much time you spend to read
your child a book, make yourself a sandwich, put a roast and veggies
in the crockpot for dinner, or compile your weekly grocery-shopping
list.

Now, imagine that while performing one of these actions, you
must find a way to survive an active shooter scenario. Not much time
to think about *and* implement an appropriate and potentially life-
saving response, is it?

But wait. You will have police and other law-enforcement personnel who can come to your aid and stop the active shooter, right?
While the answer is yes, as most areas of the United States do have
some type of contracted police coverage, the officers likely won't appear as quickly as you need them to appear to save your life before
the event is over.

## Police Response to Active Shooters

Case in point: an article published by *Police* magazine cited the Department of Homeland Security's finding that, for school shooters specifically, the average law enforcement response to these types of calls took eighteen minutes.[12] This means that the police couldn't get on scene, stop the threat, and implement life-saving measures until roughly eight minutes after shooting had already ceased. Even a five-second improvement in response time could potentially save several lives.

With more and more budget cuts to governmental agencies, this issue is likely to get worse before it gets better. For instance, on February 21, 2017, Fox 5 in San Diego, California, ran a story about how budget cuts could cause the local schools to lose twenty-one officers.[13] That's twenty-one fewer police personnel who could potentially save the lives of students and staff, leaving the entire district more vulnerable to an active shooter scenario.

In short, one cannot rely solely on police officers to stop an active shooter. Instead, it is up to all of us as individuals to do our part.

To be clear, this doesn't mean that you must always and immediately take on an active shooter one-on-one, placing your life in danger, nor should you if you can avoid it. But it *does* mean that it's your responsibility to know what you can do to better protect not only your own life but also the lives of those around you if you ever find yourself in the middle of this type of scenario and want to survive.

## *You* Are Part of the Response

That's why this nation's top law-enforcement agency suggests that you train for these types of scenarios. In their 2000 to 2013 study results, after reporting the finding that most active shooter incidents are over within a few minutes' time, the FBI stated,

Recognizing the increased active shooter threat and the swiftness with which active shooter incidents unfold, these study results support the importance of training and exercises—not only for law enforcement but also for citizens. It is important, too, that training and exercises include not only an understanding of the threats faced but also the risks and options available in active shooter incidents[14].

Basically, by regularly participating in exercises designed to mimic an active-shooter incident, you will become more prepared to respond should you find yourself in this circumstance. It's not much different than practicing how you'd escape from your home in the event of a fire or how you'd respond should a major earthquake suddenly occur. The more you practice these types of scenarios, the more efficient your response.

Since most active shooter incidents occur within ten minutes or less, it becomes *your* response that mainly determines whether you (and those around you) survive. This is especially true as, regardless of how responsive the police are, arriving on scene before the incident is over is almost impossible unless the officer was on the property or in the area when the shooting began.

## Stopping the Active Shooter

Upon hearing that innocent bystanders have a limited amount of time to formulate and implement a response, the next question is usually, "If you only have five to ten minutes from the beginning of the incident to the end, exactly *how* do you stop an active shooter?"

While some active shooter situations are ended by the shooter committing suicide (which occurs in roughly 56% of the cases) or by some type of law-enforcement response, in some of the cases, additional lives are saved by everyday people (sheepdogs) who are self-less and quick-acting enough to stop the shooter and the threat.

Specifically, in 13.1 percent of the cases studied by the FBI in 2014, it was an unarmed citizen who could safely step in and end the threat, creating a successful resolution. Half of these unarmed individuals were educators or students, which is no surprise due to the number of shootings in school-based settings during this time. The others were everyday people who happened to be in the area when the shooting began and decided to act to stop the threat.

It should be noted that in six additional cases, it was an armed person who stepped in and stopped the attack. Some were off-duty police officers or security guards. Others were citizens who were carrying a firearm. But what would have happened if those shootings had occurred in a weapon-free zone? Who would have been able to step in then?

Of course, there are also the lives saved that can't be put into numbers. After all, there's no way of knowing how many more people the shooters would have taken out had their attacks not been stopped.

Plus, there are the lives that were saved solely because someone had the forethought to create some type of obstacle or barrier that prevented the shooter from reaching and subsequently injuring or killing more victims. This happens in cases where people have overturned tables to block doors or have hidden in a dark supply closet to give the appearance that the room was empty.

## Using the 10 Minutes to Your Benefit

While it may seem like having a mere ten minutes to respond could work against you, there's a major benefit to this short time frame. Primarily, if you can manage to survive for the first ten minutes of an active killer incident, then you have a good chance of surviving the incident in its entirety.

Keep this in mind when practicing your own active shooter scenarios (whether mentally or physically), as what you do in this small-time frame could likely determine whether you survive. To better help you in your training, so you can make the situations and scenarios more realistic, or to help you if ever find yourself in this scary situation, it also helps to understand what type of person is likely to be an active shooter.

# Three

## *WHO* IS THE ACTIVE SHOOTER?

While there are no demographic groups exempt from becoming an active killer, statistically speaking, there *are* certain qualities or traits that many past shooters have shared. The first is gender.

## Male-Dominated Incidents

In the FBI's report identifying the 160 active shootings between 2000 and 2013, all the incidents involved male shooters except for six committed by females. This male-dominated trend continued in 2014 and 2015, with 39 of the 42 active shooters in those two years being male and the remaining three females.

Because more men tend to be active shooters than women, it sometimes makes it difficult to think of or remember actual cases in which females were the perpetrators of mass casualty, but these cases do occur. For example, on September 8, 2016, it was reported that five shots were fired at Alpine High School in Alpine, Texas.[15] The shooter was a fourteen-year-old girl.

In another school-based shooting, this one occurring at Louisiana Technical College, it was also a female behind the gun's trigger. In this case, the twenty-three-year-old woman reportedly killed two students and wounded twenty more before finally turning the gun on herself.[16]

## Active Shooters by Age

The FBI's statistics also reveal a little more about the age of active shooters. Here's a breakdown of the ages of the perpetrators in the shootings occurring in 2014 and 2015:

| Age Range | Number of Shooters |
|-----------|--------------------|
| Pre-Teen | 1 |
| Teen | 5 |
| 20-29 | 16 |
| 30-39 | 5 |
| 40-49 | 8 |
| 50-59 | 5 |
| 60-69 | 1 |
| 70-79 | 1 |

One look at these numbers, and you can quickly see that twenty-two of the forty-two shooters were under the age of thirty. Overall, they were responsible for more than 50 percent of the shootings.

## They Typically Work Alone

According to the FBI, out of the 40 incidents between 2014 and 2015, an overwhelming majority (38 of them) involved one active shooter per scene. The remaining two were carried out by two shooters each: a husband and a wife. And of the 160 active shooter events between 2000 and 2013, 98.9 percent of the killers acted alone. This indicates that most active shooters are solitary in this regard. In other words, they typically work alone.

This isn't always the case though. Take Columbine, for example. This incident involved two shooters: Eric Harris and Dylan Klebold.[17] So while this type of situation doesn't happen as often as the sole shooter, it can still occur.

# Additional Statistics of Interest[18]

**By The Numbers**

**40** incidents in 26 states: 20 incidents in 2014; 20 incidents in 2015.

**231** casualties: 92 killed and 139 wounded (excluding the shooters).
> *4 law enforcement officers killed and 10 wounded in 6 incidents.*[5]
> *3 unarmed security guards wounded.*

**6** incidents ended when citizens acted to end the threat. [6]

**26** incidents ended with law enforcement at the scene.

**14** incidents ended with an exchange of gunfire between the **16** shooters and law enforcement.
> *12 killed by police, one off-duty.*
> *3 committed suicide.*
> *1 surrendered to law enforcement.*

**42** shooters. [7]
> *39 male*
> *3 female.*

**2** husband-and-wife teams.

**16** shooters committed suicide.

**14** shooters were killed by law enforcement.

**12** shooters were apprehended.

## Warning Signs

Certainly, none of these demographics on their own mean that someone will someday become an active shooter. However, there are a few common signs that could potentially indicate that someone is thinking about or possibly even planning a nonrandom act of violence. These include the following:

- Aggressive or threatening behavior or remarks
- Bizarre or irrational behavior, emotional outbursts
- Sudden or extreme behavior changes
- Unresolved relationship or family issues
- Serious financial problems
- Depression or untreated mental illness and personality disorders
- Alcohol or drug abuse
- Comments or threats related to suicide
- History of violence

Keep in mind that these alone aren't usually enough to send someone over the edge, but if there are other factors (other warning signs), the person in question could be triggered to commit an act of violence.

As an example, imagine that a man you work with starts to act differently. You find out that he's going through a divorce, he just found out his wife is having an affair, or he's facing bankruptcy. As a result, he becomes depressed and starts drinking. Enough emotional stress can cause most people to crack.

## Active Shooter Triggers

Some of the time, the active shooter's trigger is work-related. Maybe the person was recently reprimanded, given a demotion at work, or forced to take a decrease in pay. Termination of employment can be a trigger as well, as can having some type of dispute with a fellow employee or with someone in a supervisory role. If the person feels like the supervisor has it out for him or her, it could easily send them over the edge.

Other times the trigger is personal. This is evidenced by the FBI's report that 10 percent of active shooter incidents are initiated with the killing of a family member. Personal situations that could serve as a catalyst for this type of event include relationship issues like going through a divorce, enduring a child-custody battle, having a child in trouble with the law, or any number of other incidents involving stress within the family unit.

Financial issues can act as a trigger as well. This is particularly huge for men because men are supposed to be the providers, to be able to take care of their families financially. When they can't, when they're forced to deal with bankruptcies, home foreclosures, or car repossessions, some just snap.

## Weapons of Choice

When we talk about the active shooter, it's pretty much implied that the shooter has some type of firearm, thanks largely to the media perpetuating the term "active shooter." Whether involving a handgun or a long gun (27 percent have used rifles, and 9 percent have used shotguns), most incidents *are* carried out with a weapon that fires a projectile. But sometimes mass killings occur with other types of weapons.

For example, edged weapons like knives and machetes have been used in the past to inflict mass amounts of bodily harm. Here are a few incidents to consider domestically and abroad:

- In 2017, a sixteen-year-old New York boy stabbed four other teens as a continuation of an in-school fight.[19]

- Four women who were identified as members of a separatist group attacked multiple innocent bystanders at a Chinese train station in 2014, ultimately killing 29 of them and causing injury to 130 others.[20]
- Twenty-two children and one adult were stabbed in a seemingly motiveless 2012 knife attack at one Chinese school.[21]
- A thirty-seven-year-old janitor with a knife killed six boys and two girls (all first or second graders) and injured fifteen more in a Japanese school in 2001, and that was after previously being arrested for accusations of "spiking the tea of four teachers" at a school in 1999.[22]
- An Australian woman who was said to suffer from "severe schizophrenia" brutally stabbed and killed all seven of her children (four sons and three daughters) and a niece in 2014.[23]
- In 2015, nine alleged Uyghur separatists killed fifty sleeping workers in a knife attack that took place at a Chinese coal mine.[24]
- Five hundred Nigerians in three different villages died at the hands of attackers with machetes in 2010 solely because they were Christian.[25]
- In 2008, Steve Kwon and his best friend attacked and killed his ex-wife, her boyfriend, her two children, and another male with a samurai sword and a bat.[26]

Other weapons used in mass killings include explosives and explosive devices. For instance, on May 28, 1927, 45 students and teachers were killed at Bath Consolidated School when more than a thousand pounds of dynamite exploded. The reason for the blast? Andrew Kehoe was upset about school-related property taxes.[27] In 2015, 22 people were killed and 120 were injured when a three-kilogram pipe bomb was detonated at a Bangkok shrine.[28]

Gasoline and matches have created their fair share of damage too. In 1990, eighty-seven people were killed at a social club that Julio Gonzalez had set on fire after having been thrown out because he was arguing with his former girlfriend. This caused the victims to be "trapped screaming and crying in the dark."[29]

Even sarin gas has been used as a mass-killing strategy. In 1995, 12 were killed and an additional 5,500 more people required treatment after ten terrorists associated with a religious cult released sarin gas in a Tokyo subway.[30]

Mass casualty can result from other objects too. For instance, in September 1911, one man entered two separate Colorado Springs homes and killed all six occupants with the blunt end of an axe.[31] (The fact that some of these incidents occurred in the early 1900s is proof that mass killings are not a new phenomenon.)

It's also not uncommon for active shooters to use more than one weapon in an attack. One piece of research conducted by the *Washington Post* found, after reviewing 130 such incidents, that "shooters brought an average of four weapons to each shooting; one carried seven guns."[32] What can drive people to this point?

# Four Primary Motives

There are many reasons that some people decide to go on mass-killing sprees, but they can all be boiled down to four main motives: anger or revenge, mental illness or a personality disorder, ideological reasons, or criminal intent.

### ANGER OR REVENGE

If something happens that causes a person to feel angry, he or she may decide to get revenge via an active shooting. Causes of this anger could include job termination, having conflict with someone, or dealing with financial and/or personal relationship issues. Having been bullied or humiliated could also elicit this response if the person believes that violence will solve the issue because they believe others are to blame. One example of a revenge-type shooting occurred in a Bay District school-board meeting in Florida; the incident was captured entirely on video, which I show in my training.

When the meeting was opened to public comment, so citizens could voice their concerns, fifty-six-year-old Clay Duke got up, spray-painted a red *V* in a circle on the wall, and then kicked all the spectators out, leaving only the board members in the room. They had no choice but to listen to Duke express his anger at the fact that his wife (who had previously worked for the district) had been fired and at the financial issues that were created, all while he continued to wave a gun.[33]

After moments of some back-and-forth conversation and comments, Duke aimed directly at superintendent Bill Husfelt and fired. This was followed by several shots fired at the other board members as well. It was then that Mike Jones, a retired police officer and the school's chief of security, entered the room and shot and wounded Duke, ultimately causing Duke to commit suicide with his own gun.

Duke wanted revenge on the school board for what he felt "they'd done" to his wife and ultimately to him. In his eyes, they were to blame for the way his life had taken a downward spiral, so they became the target of his retribution.

### MENTAL ILLNESS OR PERSONALITY DISORDER

Have you ever looked at a picture of someone who committed a mass killing, like James Eagan Holmes (who dressed in tactical clothing, set off teargas grenades, and shot into the audience with multiple firearms inside a Century 16 movie theater in Aurora, Colorado, during a midnight screening of the film *The Dark Knight Rises*) or Adam Lanza (the active shooter at Sandy Hook Elementary in Newtown, Connecticut, who caused the death of twenty first graders and six school staff in 2012)?[34] Could you see it in their eyes that something was amiss? This often happens in cases in which mental illness or personality disorder is the underlying cause of the random act of violence.

The National Alliance on Mental Illness (NAMI) reports that one out of every five (or 43.8 million) Americans suffer from some type of mental illness per year.[35] Additionally, 18.1 percent of these types of disorders involve anxiety, 6.9 percent involve depression, 2.6 percent involve bipolar disorder, and 1.1 percent involve schizophrenia. Certainly, most people with mental disorders don't strive to kill masses of people, but sometimes these mental conditions are a contributing factor.

Take the Virginia Tech shooter Seung Hui Cho, for instance. Prior to killing thirty-two people and wounding seventeen others on April 16, 2017, Cho created a pre-shooting videotape confession in which he said, "I did it. I had to." He also took twenty-nine different photos of himself in a wide array of positions, many of which involved him pointing a gun directly at the camera. It was later discovered that Cho's medical records revealed a history of mental-health issues; Cho had even been admitted to a psych ward in 2005 after his roommate said that he had threatened suicide.[36]

## IDEOLOGICAL REASONS

Some active shooters commit these violent acts with the intention of creating fear within the population, what we commonly refer to as "terror," based on a cause that they care or feel deeply about. Sometimes the cause is political, sometimes it's religious or racial, or sometimes it's something completely different in which that the person is still extremely passionate.

An example of extreme religion-based mass killings in modern-day times are the murders attributed to ISIS, the Islamic State in Iraq and Syria. On July 16, 2016, the *New York Times* published data from a self-conducted analysis indicating that more than 1,200 people outside Iraq and Syria have died at the hands of ISIS, almost half of whom were Westerners.[37] Of course, that doesn't include the time 2,977 people were killed by another radical Islamic group, Al Qaeda, in the 9/11 attacks (2,753 of whom were on one of the hijacked planes or in the twin towers, 184 of whom died when the plane crashed into the Pentagon, and 40 of whom were passengers and crew members killed when their plane crashed into a Pennsylvania field).[38]

Ideological reasons were also behind the 2009 mass killing committed at Fort Hood by US Army Psychiatrist Major Nidal Malik Hasan. Based on reports, it's said that Hasan shouted "Allahu Akbar"—which translates to "God is great" in Arabic—before killing one Department of Defense employee and twelve service members.[39]

An example of an active killer whose racial ideology was the foundation of his ruthless acts is Dylann Roof, a twenty-one-year-old self-proclaimed white supremacist, who, on June 17, 2015, initiated a mass shooting against an all-black congregation at Emanuel African Methodist Episcopal Church in downtown Charleston, South Carolina, with the hope of starting a race war. After killing nine people and injuring one other, he escaped but was apprehended a short while later and was ultimately convicted and sentenced to death.[40]

## CRIMINAL INTENT

The fourth reason someone would plan and execute a mass killing is that the person is simply a ruthless criminal. In these cases, the event usually begins with a criminal act and evolves from there. There have been countless reports of robbers taking employees and patrons of cafés, liquor, and other retail stores to the back room and, even after cleaning out the store safe, killing everyone execution style.

A specific representation of this type of scenario is the North Hollywood shootout that took place on February 28, 1997. It was on this day that two bank robbers, Larry Phillips and Emil Matasareanu—wearing masks and homemade body armor and carrying assault rifles—spent forty-four harrowing minutes in a shootout with police.[41]

Essentially, what started out as a bank robbery (a criminal act) ended with more than a thousand rounds being sent out into the streets of Hollywood that day. Fortunately, the only ones who lost their lives were the shooters, although eleven officers and seven innocent bystanders were injured in the attack.

## DUAL MOTIVES

In some active shooter cases, there are two reasons behind the attack, which means there was a dual cause. This was the case with twenty-two-year-old Elliot Rodger, the gunman behind the University of California, Santa Barbara, attack on May 23, 2014, that left six dead and fourteen wounded. In a video that Rodger shot prior to the killings, he shared how he felt overwhelmingly rejected by women (even revealing that he was a virgin who'd never been kissed), so his goal was revenge.

If you watch Rodger as he states that "tomorrow is the day of retribution, the day in which I will have my revenge against humanity,"[42] you can clearly see that something is mentally amiss, primarily when he shares his intent to kill, followed by an evil laugh. Clinical psychologist Dr. David Gustaf Thompson weighed in on Rodger's mental health, saying he wasn't surprised at the video's contents because, while the case was "more extreme than most,"[43] it's one he sees quite often with individuals who have been coddled emotionally.

Rodger also spoke in great detail about the attention he'd wanted but never received. The shooting was how he was finally going to get that attention; he was going to take control.

Another example of dual motives is seen in the case when, on June 12, 2016, twenty-nine-year-old Omar Mateen walked into Pulse, a gay nightclub in Orlando, Florida, and killed forty-nine people and wounded fifty-eight others. Though he'd sworn allegiance to ISIS (acting out of religious ideology), he targeted the homosexual community, even though he was allegedly gay himself.[44]

## It's All about Control

In the end, whether the incident is initiated due to anger, revenge, ideology, mental illness, or criminal behavior, the primary driving factor behind active shooter incidents is control. This control gives shooters the sense of power they long for after feeling powerless to change the factors or events in their lives that have brought them to this point. Shooters are attempting to take charge when it feels like they don't have any control or need more control over what is occurring in their lives. You see this all the time in cases in which shooters have been previously bullied by student peers or supervisors, were belittled for their beliefs, were rejected by their wives, or were otherwise in situations that they couldn't change or rectify rationally.

The active shooter knows that engaging in this type of event gives them ultimate control, ultimate power. They control others via fear and the taking of their lives. They also gain (or regain) control over their own lives. Some in my industry call this the "God complex." You will read many times over the course of this book that the primary goal of active killers is to kill as many people as possible in as short a time as possible because they know that the end *will* come, so they need to achieve their goal quickly. And even in death, they will have control because most active killers take their own lives before anyone else has the opportunity. See the chronological list of active killers who took their own lives, from 2000 to 2017, at the end of this book to illustrate how frequently they would rather kill themselves than lose the sense of control and power they have, in their minds, regained from their horrible deeds. The exception to this however, are those who kill in the name of Islam. Radical Muslims believe they will live forever in "paradise" if they die while advancing or defending the name of Allah and the religion of Islam. Escaping to fight again or fighting to the death is their preferred conclusion, as witnessed during and after the Inland Regional Center killings in San Bernardino, California.

And of course, in the eyes of the killers, the best way to enhance getting the control they always wanted is to keep the control after the event by letting the world know who they are and that they have control. Many active shooters, such as Elliot Rodger in Santa Barbara and Seung-Hui Cho at Virginia Tech, knew their story would be publicized, allowing that control to last even beyond their death. Those two went as far as creating videos of themselves describing what they would do prior to their killing spree, so the media could perpetuate their brutal acts long after they were gone. Unfortunately, this has given would-be killers a study guide to plan future attacks; they now know their stories will live on long past their demise.

## What They Fear and What They Don't

Active shooters don't generally fear death. Yes, they may fear dying at the hands of another because it takes control away from them, but they usually have no fear of death itself. In fact, if you've ever seen a recorded active shooter incident, you may have noticed that the shooter had a tremendous sense of calm before and during the attack. This is because they felt in control. It's bizarre and hard to comprehend as a normal thinking person, but all witness accounts speak to that.

The one thing the active shooter *does* fear is not accomplishing his or her goal of killing as many people as possible in as short a time as possible. That's why they're intent on taking out as many people as they can as quickly as they can. To be stopped short would mean they didn't do what they set out to do; it would mean they lost control.

So how do you deal with individuals with this type of faulty mindset, with these "wolves"? It all begins with creating the right mindset yourself: a survival mindset.

# Four

## SECURITY AND SURVIVAL MINDSETS

While there are many definitions that explain exactly what mindset is, the one that best relates to the mindset needed to survive an active shooter is "a fixed mental attitude or disposition that predetermines a person's responses to, and interpretations of, situations."[45] What does this mean in real-life terms, and, perhaps more importantly, why does it matter so much in this scenario?

Put simply, it is your mindset (the way you think) that will predetermine how you'll react in each situation. Thus, if you want to react effectively if you ever find yourself face-to-face with an active shooter, creating this type of life-saving reaction begins with your thoughts.

For example, if you believe that the only way to effectively settle a disagreement with your spouse is to give in and say that you're wrong—even when you don't believe you are—then that is exactly what you'll do. Conversely, if you feel that marital arguments can only be settled when you stand your ground and never give in, then that's what you'll do instead. Both are examples of predetermined reactions.

## Security Mindset

Having a security mindset should be part of your everyday life. Whether you're going out in public to go grocery shopping for your family or to present a new or innovative business idea to a room full of conference attendees, you should be thinking about how secure the area is, as well as how you'd respond if someone breached that security. In the military and law enforcement, this is referred to as "situational awareness."

This is extremely important because active shooters like crowded places with lots of people. (Remember that their goal is to kill as many people as quickly as they possibly can.) For them, it's like shooting fish in a barrel. They have the advantage.

A notable example of this is the active shootings that occur at places of worship. In fact, a very busy time for my security company is during the high holy days for the Jewish population because synagogues become major targets, so they need extra protection from individuals who are intent on doing them harm.

## Survival Mindset

In an active shooter scenario, how you feel about survival plays a critical role in whether that's what you'll do. In other words, it isn't necessarily that one type of response is better than another, but the action *you* choose in that situation is based on your interpretation of what's happening and what you believe is the right thing to do. Your actions ultimately mirror your beliefs.

This underscores the importance of having a survival mindset in active shooter scenarios. When you have your own safety and security in mind, as well as the safety and security of those around you, you are telling your mind how to respond in that type of situation. You are telling it that your survival comes first, so your mind and body had better act accordingly.

Creating this mindset first involves becoming aware of what is happening in your immediate surroundings, so your mind recognizes the fact that it needs to formulate an appropriate reaction—a reaction that could potentially save your life, as well as the lives of your family, friends, coworkers, or anyone else in your immediate vicinity.

Having this alert mindset makes you more prepared. It helps you plan for how you'll respond to an incident, should it occur, because it makes you think about the incident *before* it happens. This keeps you from freezing and doing nothing in a violent encounter, which is the one response that will likely get you killed.

## Fight, Flight, or Freeze

When you're faced with a life-or-death situation, your body will have one of three possible reactions. It will either want to fight, flee, or freeze. Fight is when you decide to take on the attacker one-on-one, determined to overpower him or her, so that if anyone survives the event, it is going to be you.

The second option is flight; this is when you escape the dangerous situation. For example, if you're leaving the mall and approach your car only to find someone hiding nearby and ready to attack, you run away before giving the attacker the chance. You evade the situation, so your attacker can't execute his or her plan.

The third possible response is the most dangerous, and that is to freeze. This is when you are completely paralyzed and unable to move, which also means that you can't fight off the attacker, *and* you're unable to flee. This makes you a sitting duck for the person intent on doing you harm, which is the worst possible place to find yourself in.

A notable example of this occurred during the incident mentioned earlier, when an armed man walked into a school-board meeting to take revenge for the fact that his wife was fired. In one video I show during my presentations, you see that once the first shot is fired by the intended assailant, only one board member dives under the boardroom desk to use cover and concealment to survive the event. Most of the people being shot at simply freeze, even after several minutes of hearing from the armed man himself that he is going to kill them, in shock at what is occurring with no predetermined reaction to save themselves.

So how do you get the type of mindset that enables you to respond appropriately in an active shooter scenario, so you don't freeze, increasing your chances of survival? You begin to think with your survival in mind.

## The Pollyanna Effect

The Pollyanna effect literally means a subconscious bias toward the positive, which some could even label as denial. Admittedly, there are lots of Pollyannas in this world. These are the people who have a tough time seeing the bad side of humanity because they're always looking at the positives in life; they are the sheep, who find it difficult to see or predict when someone is intent on committing harm.

Overall, this isn't a bad thing because it means that you have empathy, that you're able to see beyond a person's bad behavior when that behavior isn't necessarily their intent. However, if this is you, you may also struggle with creating a security mindset.

As a Pollyanna, you don't want to see the evil in this world. But the problem with this mindset is that because there *is* evil in this world, you are left completely unprepared and unable to recognize when you find yourself looking at someone who doesn't fit in or looks threatening. You can't easily see the potential problem because you only want to see the good.

Ultimately, this mindset will work against you. Not that I'm saying you should completely change the way you think, because I'm not. I'm saying that this is how some people think, and it has gotten them injured or killed as a result, so adding a security mindset to your precognitive ideology can keep you alive. That's why it helps to be suspicious when appropriate and to listen to your gut.

## Listen to Your Gut

In his book *The Gift of Fear: Survival Signals That Protect Us from Violence*, author Gavin DeBecker demonstrates how every individual should learn to trust the inherent "gift" of their gut instinct and how this physical response already exists in everyone, making it possible to avoid potential trauma and harm by learning to recognize various warning signs and precursors to violence[46].

I liken fear to your body's other natural early-warning systems, like hunger, thirst, and fatigue. When you're hungry, you know that you need fuel. When you're thirsty, there's no denying that if you don't get water within the necessary amount of time, you could perish. And when your body runs out of the necessary energy resources it needs to go on, it must rest and recharge.

Basically, your stomach acts as your second brain. It tells you when it may be necessary to become more alert and hyperaware if you want to survive. While you never allow yourself to become consumed by this gut reaction, you do need to listen to it. You need to pay attention and heed its warning when it tells you that something just doesn't feel right.

When you feel fear, like when you're in a dark alley or an unfamiliar environment at night with limited visibility and suddenly feel the hair stand up on the back of your neck, yet no one's in sight, your body and your mind are telling you to be on high alert. Something is amiss, even if you can't quite put your finger on what.

My dad was a master at this. As a former law-enforcement officer and the founder of our company, he watched people and, more often than not, they were not a potential threat. But he did realize when people didn't fit in, which is when his level of alertness was piqued. As a result, no one put anything over on my dad because he was always ready. He was always situationally aware.

## Developing Situational Awareness

An extreme example of situational awareness is the character Jason Bourne in the Bourne series. In one scene of the movie *The Bourne Identity*, Bourne and his female companion are sitting in a restaurant, and he is explaining to her how he sees everything, so he begins talking about the first thing he noticed when he came into the restaurant. He shares how he was "catching sidelines" and "looking for the exit."

Bourne goes on to reveal that he could tell her the license-plate numbers of all six cars in the parking lot and that he knows the best place to look for a gun is in the cab of the gray truck outside. He knows that "the waitress is left-handed, and the guy at the counter weighs 215 pounds and knows how to handle himself"; he knows every other detail he's picked up on that could potentially help him if confronted by a threat. He even says he knows his own personal physical response, stating that "at this altitude, I can run flat out for half a mile before my hands start to shake[47]."

You want to train your mind to react to situations with this type of detail and clarity, so you're 100% prepared should they occur. Okay, maybe not as prepared as Bourne, but you get the point. This is something I call being "proactively reactionary."

## Proactive Reactionism

Proactive reactionism is a term I created, so you won't find it in any dictionary. What it involves is the idea that you can train yourself to react appropriately to something you've never experienced if you prepare your mind in advance.

This type of proactive physical and mental reaction works because you

1. imagine a scenario before it happens;
2. have a plan for that scenario; and
3. make the plan become second nature.

So how does this work? How does this type of training translate into a positive response to an active shooter situation?

In times of stress, you default to your level of training. For instance, in one study, people were interviewed after performing the Heimlich maneuver or CPR to save someone's life, and, when asked how they knew how to do it, they responded that they didn't know but had had training years ago, and it just came back to them in that instant. Their minds defaulted to the training that they had had and immediately began the steps necessary when the time came, moving that knowledge from the back (subconscious) of their minds to the front, ultimately making it possible to save the person's life.

It's kind of the same principle as riding a bike. You may go ten, twenty, or thirty years without placing your butt on a bicycle seat, but once you do, you might be a little rusty, but you pick right up where you left off. The same is true regarding training in active shooter scenarios. Once you internalize and tell your body how to respond, that's likely what it'll do if you're ever confronted with someone who is intent on doing you harm.

Some people are taught these types of responses from childhood. For instance, as I have stated, I had a father who was in law enforcement, so I witnessed his behavior and often emulated it naturally. But if you weren't raised that way or didn't have that example when you were growing up, let me assure you that it's never too late to learn. Survival can *easily* become your first reaction, your fixed mindset. But the understanding of exactly how to survive has changed over time, which is why I created the ALIVE Active Shooter Survival Plan.

ALIVE Active Shooter Survival Plan

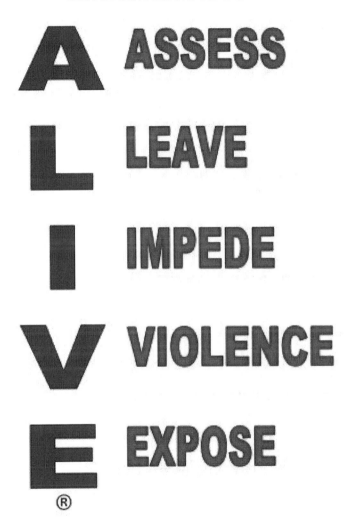

A  ASSESS

L  LEAVE

I  IMPEDE

V  VIOLENCE

E  EXPOSE

# Five

## ASSESS

When faced with an active killer situation, the first thing you want to do is assess the situation: stop, breathe, and think about what may be happening around you. This helps keep you from panicking, continues the steady flow of oxygen to your brain, and allows you to respond in a way that will maximize your safety while putting your response plan into action.

The worst possible time to create a plan is when you're in the middle of a crisis. That would be like not thinking about how you'd escape your second-floor bedroom in the event of a fire, yet waking up one night to flames in the only stairwell in your house. Your failure to plan could easily mean you don't make it out alive. At a minimum, it will raise your stress level and delay your response as you try to quickly think about your options while the flames grow closer and closer.

This is also why training with active killer scenarios is important. The more you know how you want to respond before you need to, the more you're able to respond calmly and rationally, and the better your response will be. Furthermore, the better your response is, the greater your likelihood of survival.

## Visualization: Creating a Plan *Before* You Need It

Visualization exercises help a lot in this type of situation as they allow you to create a mental plan. They walk you through many different scenarios and force you to think about what could possibly happen. They also set the stage for you to plan your response, so if you're ever faced with someone intent on taking your life, you'll know exactly what to do.

Another benefit of visualization is that while you can't possibly physically train for every potential violent encounter in your life, you *can* train mentally very easily because all you need is your imagination and a little bit of free time. Visualization is extremely effective too. In fact, this is a technique that many law-enforcement and other public-safety responders are taught early in their careers as a way of increasing their safety when responding to what are sometimes harrowing situations.

This simple visualization works by imagining a scenario in which you're faced with an active killer. As you envision this event unfolding before you, mentally walk yourself through a successful response.

When performing your visualization, run through the scenario multiple times until it feels like you have your response down pat. Then, once you're comfortable with your response, change the scenario. This forces you to consider other alternatives and modify your plan accordingly. For instance, imagine the killer entering through a different door, carrying a different weapon, or even looking physically different. The more possible plans you have in place, the more readily available and better you will respond.

Ideally, you want to use as many of your senses as you can while visualizing. This makes the situation as realistic to your mind as possible, and the more your brain feels like you're in an actual encounter, the better equipped it will be to carry out your plan when needed.

For example, let's say you imagine an active killer entering your workplace. If this happens, what noises are you likely to hear?

Machines humming? Coworkers screaming? What stands between you and the killer? A Plexiglas window? Nothing? What limits will you have to your sight that could put you in harm's way? Is your view blocked by a cabinet or file shelves? Are you in a cubicle or your own office? Are there locks on your door? Your goal is to try to imagine the scenario as realistically as you can.

## Think of Your Plan

If you suddenly realize that you're in an active killer scenario, it is during the assessment phase that you want to think about which plan to put into action. Thus, you'll need to consider your plan as it relates to the incident. Think about your options as they relate to your plan.

For instance, will you be able to safely and effectively leave the area, or are you going to have to stay and fight? If you must fight, what objects are in your vicinity that you could use as weapons? Is anyone there who could help you overpower and take down the attacker or attackers?

All in all, you want to think about your plan and assess your situation before you act. Your only goal at this point is to determine which of your next actions are most appropriate. Think about what is happening around you and about your options in relation to the events.

## Don't Just Run

While it may be tempting or second nature to just take off running, that may be the *last* thing you want to do. What you think might be the right direction to go—a way out—may take you into the center of the incident instead.

The better approach, the safer approach, is to be methodical. If you do move, move briskly, but when you come to a corner or any other area that impairs your line of sight, peek around it first to see what's on the other side. Don't just move blindly and hope for the best.

Even though you may be hearing sounds coming from one direction, that doesn't necessarily tell you which way safety lies. Halls tend to echo, and the acoustics can be deceiving, so you might not be able to tell the killer's location based on the noises you're hearing.

Pause and assess for a split second to gather your thoughts and take control of your conscious next steps. Give your brain that moment it needs to let whatever is happening sink in, so you can consider your full situation and surroundings before deciding what to do next.

## Isn't Pausing Dangerous?

I once had a guy challenge the idea of pausing and assessing in one of my trainings by saying, "But if you wait three seconds, the guy might come there and kill you." Maybe you've even had this very same thought yourself. If so, let's clear this up right now.

I assure you that when your adrenaline hits, which it *will* in an active killer situation, you can think about five minutes' worth of thoughts in three seconds. If you've ever been in a life-or-death situation, then you already know that this is true. Your mind will go faster than you've ever thought possible.

So, taking a quick moment to fully realize the situation around you isn't going to slow you down because it's going to be happening at faster-than-normal speeds. Besides, you must pause and let your mind go through these motions because if you don't, you'll likely forgo rational thought and react emotionally or freak out, a response that can easily result in your making the wrong decision.

## Prepare to Kill or Be Killed

When you're assessing the situation, this is also the time to start ramping yourself up mentally, preparing your mind to either kill or be killed. You need to be ready to take some type of action, no matter what that action is, to save your own life and possibly even the lives of those around you.

This is a difficult concept for some people, but it's one that is necessary if you want to survive. Remember that the active killer's goal is to take out as many people as quickly as possible. He or she doesn't care that you have a family, an excellent job, or a lot to live for. All he or she cares about is ending your life before moving on to the next victim, and the next.

That's why your assessment of the situation, of your options as they relate to your specific incident, should include formulating the attitude that if anyone is going home today, it's going to be you. You need to decide at the very beginning of the event that you'll do whatever is necessary to protect your life.

Once you've assessed the situation and reaffirmed in your mind that you'll take as much action as is necessary to survive the incident, it's time to move on to the next step. This involves deciding whether it's an option for you to leave.

# Six

## LEAVE

It's often said that the best fight is the one that's avoided, and this rings especially true in active killer incidents. Because the attacker's primary goal is to kill as many people as possible as quickly as possible, if you can get away and escape to a safe area, then that's by far the best thing you can do.

There was a time when "lockdown" was the first response to a report of criminal activity or a sighting of a predator or active shooter around schools, but we have learned that we will likely not know about active killers until after they have already entered the building. If this were the case, locking down may be the worst response if leaving the area is possible.

## Get Away from the Threat—Fast!

Get as far away from the threat as quickly as you possibly can. This means that once you've assessed the situation, decided which plan to put into action, and determined your most viable and accessible escape route, you want to *run like hell* as far away as you can.

43

Even if you're not in the best physical shape possible, push your legs to move you as fast as they humanly can. The adrenaline released by your system will help, enabling you to go quicker than you would under normal, non-stressful circumstances.

Don't stop running until you're someplace where the killer can't see you. Depending on your location and the incident, this may involve heading to a neighboring business or building, going to your vehicle, or finding some other place that is well out of the killer's vicinity.

Obviously, the distance you must go to be considered safe is going to be determined by the type of weapon the active killer is using. However, remember that, in most cases, the active killers bring *several* different weapons to the incident. So, don't just assume that he or she only has one. Run as if there are several weapons, and don't stop running until you're as far away as you can safely go.

## Notify Those around You

In addition to getting yourself out of the area, you also want to notify everyone in your immediate vicinity of control about what you believe might be happening. Share with them that it's possible an active killer is near you, so you need to go, and you need to go *now*!

If they've had this training too (which is highly possible if they're one of your coworkers and attended one of my survival classes sponsored by your company), they'll know exactly what to do. That's why I always recommend that everyone in an organization have an opportunity to attend the training. The more you can work as a group, the more effective your response.

If they haven't had this training, be ready to tell them exactly what they must do. This is important because without proper training, they may want to do something that could inevitably put you and them in greater harm. You can help prevent that by giving some direction.

When notifying others that they need to go, you must have a command presence. What this means is that you need to be assertive, to take control. There's usually one person in every group who will automatically step into this role (sheepdogs), but if your group doesn't have one, then that person needs to be you.

Yell at those around you if necessary: "Get out now!" or "Run as far and as fast as you can!" Be firm and direct. Sound like you mean business, using the same tone of voice you would if you saw a young child reaching for a hot stove. Then, as a group, leave the area of danger and don't stop running until you are too far away to be harmed.

## When You're Responsible for Others

If you're responsible for others, you want to usher them with commanding urgency as well. This could occur in incidents if you're a day-care provider or a teacher at a school. As a nurse on a hospital ward, you'd be responsible for your patients, and as a hotel manager, you're responsible for your guests.

If you're an employer or someone who is in a supervisory role, then you're responsible for your staff. Take charge and use authority when telling them to leave. If you must, direct them where to go. If the group requires it, such as may occur if you're responsible for a second-grade class or individuals with disabilities, then you may also need to lead the way.

Think about these things when visualizing your plan. The more you know what to do beforehand, the easier it will be for you to keep your calm while establishing control.

Where is the best place to direct them to go or to go yourself if you're on your own?

## Where to Go

If the incident is occurring inside a building, and you can exit that building, run as far away as possible. Again, the more distance you can put between you and the killer, the better off you are.

If you can't get out, or if it's closer than getting out, run to a secure location (or a safe room). Ideally, this is a room where you can lock and barricade the door. It's also a room with either a small window or no window at all, or a window that can somehow be blocked off, so the killer can't see inside if he or she makes it that far.

The best safe rooms are also rooms that can stop or dramatically slow down flying bullets. For instance, if there's a room available that has block walls and one that has just drywall, the room with block walls is your better option because the walls have more stopping power.

Whether you leave the area entirely or go to a safe room, leave your belongings behind. Well, most of them, anyway.

## Leave (Most of) Your Belongings Behind

If you've ever flown, then you've probably heard one of the flight attendants give the pre-takeoff speech. And if you've listened to it, then you already know that in it they explain that, in the event of a water landing, you're to leave all your belongings behind and just focus on getting yourself off the plane.

That makes sense, right? Can you imagine how long it would take to evacuate everyone if all the passengers went for their carry-ons first? Or what if you were denied access to one of the rafts because there wasn't any more room, yet it was half full of luggage?

The same advice applies here for the same general reasons. Gathering your things will delay your escape, and the last thing you want is a large purse or briefcase weighing you down when you're trying to evade an active killer. But there are two exceptions to this rule.

First, if you have a weapon with you, such as if you're registered to legally carry a concealed firearm in your state, then you want to take that with you if you can get access to it quickly and safely. This way, you'll have it if you are forced to fight; your weapon isn't going to do you any good if you've left it behind.

Many law-enforcement representatives would argue that a civilian having a gun in this situation is ill-advised, if for no other reason than officer safety. I understand and appreciate this school of thought. However, as someone who grew up with guns and has trained with and used them on several occasions, I believe that if I have a gun, I'm taking it with me! Just be sure to keep your weapon hidden unless you need it and to drop it immediately when confronted by law enforcement. Remember that the responding officers aren't going to know who the good guys are and who the bad guys are; you don't want them to mistake you for the shooter.

The second thing you'll want to take with you is your cell phone. This enables you to call 911 *while you're exiting*, which is critical because a faster law-enforcement response can reduce the time frame of the killing incident.

A response that is five seconds faster not only saves the lives of potential victims but also means the killer will be stopped more quickly. Law enforcement will detain the active killer alive or kill him or her to stop the threat, or the killer will take his or her own life.

In these scenarios, the result is the same. The threat is over, and your actions regarding leaving the scene helped you, and maybe others, survive the incident.

If you're not able to leave, it becomes necessary to do something else—and the next best response is to impede the active killer.

# Seven

## IMPEDE

Impeding an active killer means that you need to do everything possible to limit his or her opportunity and ability to get to you. Your goal is to be so difficult to reach that it's not even worth it to the killer to try.

The reason this works to your advantage is that in most instances, killers will take the path of least resistance. This makes sense since their goal is to do as much damage and take as many lives as they can in as little time as possible. Therefore, they're not going to spend a lot of time trying to get you if you make yourself a hard target, which is precisely why you want to be difficult to get to and difficult to find.

In a situation where you are in an open area and unable to barricade yourself in a room or to find an area that is difficult to access, impeding may not be possible. To make yourself a hard target, you need to find cover, or at least something that's going to conceal you. What's the difference?

## Cover versus Concealment

Concealment basically means that you're hidden from view. For instance, if you stood behind a black shower curtain in a dark bathroom, you'd be concealed as anyone who walked by the room wouldn't see you there.

Cover, on the other hand, is an object that not only hides you from view but also would likely stop a bullet or other projectile weapon from reaching and striking you (which a shower curtain would not do). Good examples of cover include a thick wooden table, a sturdy bookshelf loaded with books, or the engine block of a car.

If you've ever played paintball, it's likely that you already know the difference between concealment and cover. Cover will stop the paintball from striking you, hitting whatever is between you and the shooter. Concealment means that even if the shooter couldn't see you, you're probably going to be walking away with a big, fat welt.

When an active shooter event unfolds, look around you and take in your surroundings to find the best place to go, the place that is out of eyesight of the active shooter or killer. The safer the area where you decide to hunker down, the better your chances of survival.

Ideally, you want to find cover, just in case you find yourself in the killer's line of fire. But that's not always possible. Sometimes you are only presented with the option of concealing yourself, which is certainly better than nothing at all.

When I was a kid growing up in Colorado, my friends and I would battle each other using BB guns. (I know, brilliant, right?) We knew we had to keep ourselves away from our "enemies," so knowing where they were at all times was essential to avoiding getting shot.

In a situation where an active shooter is in an open location with multiple targets, he will almost always aim at the closest and most easily accessible target. It's your objective to remain hidden, if the shooter doesn't already know where you are, or behind cover, making it more difficult to hit you. However, the shooter will likely be walking around looking for new targets, so you still need to know where the shooter is and adjust your position or cover to avoid becoming a victim.

A childhood BB-gun war is a very simplified example, but the principles of evasion are the same. You are still in a situation where someone's intent is to hit you with a projectile, so your objective is to stay out of view and/or make it difficult to hit you. This means that you'll need to be aware of the shooter's position as much as possible.

And if you do find your way to a room, there are many things you can do once there to impede the killer and make yourself a more difficult target. One option is to *lock and block*.

## Lock and Block

Lock and block refers to the process you want to follow when securing the door, so the killer cannot get through it and gain access to the room.

The first part is simply a reminder to lock the door if you can. Sometimes this alone is enough to stop a killer from entering because either he or she thinks the room is empty *or* you've made it harder to get at you, so the killer moves on to other, easier targets.

Sadly, lots of companies I present this response plan to don't even have locks on their conference-room doors, which is unfortunate because this is a very simple fix that could potentially save lives.

The second part of the lock-and-block process involves blocking the door, so the killer cannot easily gain entry. Even if the door *does* lock, you should still take this additional step to better protect yourself and anyone else in the room.

If the door has a window in it, block that off as well. Lots of door windows have shades that you can pull to disrupt the view, which is what I recommend when consulting with business owners and managers who would like to improve the safety of their businesses.

If your door doesn't have a shade or a blind, then just find something to cover it. Pieces of paper taped up, a curtain pulled from an outside window, or even your shirt or jacket will often do the trick.

Using lock and block slows the shooter down, so he or she will likely pass that door to pursue other targets. It also keeps the shooter from seeing who is inside and shooting into the room.

You must place your cell phone on silent when you're locked and blocked in a room, so that incoming texts and calls don't draw the killer's attention. If the news is already broadcasting the event, or others are aware of what is transpiring, you will likely begin getting texts and calls from friends and loved ones to find out if you are all right. The last thing you want is that cell phone going off just as a shooter has decided to bypass your location because he or she believes no one is present.

Remember: your goal if you're unable to leave the area is to be difficult to find and to secure your location as best you can.

## Notify

If possible, you should have already notified emergency services. But if you couldn't do that and must now hide and remain quiet, many law-enforcement agencies now have the capability to receive notification of an emergency through text message using text-to-911, so you can advise dispatch of the situation and communicate with them as the scene unfolds. They will be able to relay information to you from their officers, so you may be able to escape if the shooter has moved to the other side of the building.

There are also public-announcement applications for smartphones, frequently used on college campuses now, that will not only notify you of the presence of an active killer but also advise you as the situation progresses. You will see more and more of these technological advances to aid in active shooter survival used in educational and health-care facilities and in businesses.

There may even be times when someone is able to advise you using an audible public-announcement system to notify you where the shooter is and the status of the event.

## Better Securing the Door

There are a couple of ways to better secure the door to the room, regardless of whether it locks or not. For instance, if it opens in, and you don't have some type of intruder-defense device (which I recommend all businesses acquire and conduct drills with), you can use a simple door wedge to prevent it from opening. When using a door wedge (the type used to stop an opened door from closing), it must have the appropriate bottom to work with the flooring in your facility. A hard wedge on a tile floor would not be as effective as a rubber wedge on carpet, but it can still work. To reinforce its effectiveness, you could place your foot behind the wedge but keep your body very low or to the side of the door in the event the shooter tries shooting through the door.

Another way is to block the door with everything possible, putting the heaviest items against it first. If you block the door physically with your body, again, stay low and close to the door or off to the side to avoid shots if the killer has a gun and decides to fire in your direction.

If the door opens out (like doors that have a scissor arm at the top), and you don't have a predesigned intruder-defense device, you can always use a belt to keep the scissors together, making it more difficult to open. If you don't have a belt, use an extension cord or anything else you can find to constrict the door closer.

You can also secure the handle on an outward-opening door, so it can't easily be pulled open. This can be accomplished with a belt or any other item that you can latch onto and either hold or secure to something else in the room. Again, even if the door does open out, you still want to block it with everything possible, placing the heaviest items closest to the door itself. Having access to a safe room can be a tremendous advantage in surviving an active killer event.

## Qualities of a Practical but Adequate Safe Room

For a room to be considered sufficiently safe during an active killer incident but still practical enough to not be excessive in an office environment, it should have the following qualities: The most basic safe room is simply a closet, copy room, or internal conference room with the hollow-core door replaced with an exterior-grade solid-core door that has a dead bolt and longer hinge screws and strike-plate screws to resist battering. Sometimes the ceiling is reinforced or gated to prevent easy access from an attic, overhead crawl space, or drop ceiling.

More expensive safe rooms have walls and a door reinforced with sheets of steel, Kevlar, or bullet-resistant fiberglass. The hinges and strike plate are often reinforced with long screws. Some safe rooms may also have externally vented ventilation systems and a separate telephone connection. They might also connect to an escape shaft. Rooms like this are often expensive and therefore not common in a corporate environment.

Any room intended to be utilized as a safe room in the case of a violent attack should have a video intercom, like those made by BEC Integrated Systems or Docooler for less than $200, so people inside the room can see and hear who is outside. This way, innocent people can be seen and verified when trying to enter the room, and the attacker's actions and whereabouts can be monitored.

Being aware of these types of qualities can help you pick the safest room possible, especially if the incident occurs someplace you're familiar with, like at work. This enables you to preselect the rooms you'd go to, if possible, during an active killer incident.

Secondarily, if you own a business or are somehow responsible for employee safety, you can build a safe room into your office plans. If your building or space is already established, you can still modify certain areas to make them safer for your staff and anyone else who may be visiting your facility.

## What Hide Does *Not* Mean

During the Columbine incident, several of the kids got under their desks to attempt to hide. The problem with this type of response is that the two shooters could easily identify their victims. They essentially became easy targets because not only were they not behind cover, they weren't even really concealed.

For this reason, it has become imperative to teach students the difference between hiding under their desks or tables and hiding in a place that provides effective cover and concealment, depending on the event. In the case of a violent attack, this way of hiding simply makes them sitting ducks. Old reaction methods are not effective in modern-day active killer scenarios. Instead, innovative approaches need to be created, and one of them is to not just hide, but to hide in a spot that gives you the best chance of survival.

Regardless of how well you hide, though, sometimes it's just not enough. Sometimes you're faced with no other option but to be violent and fight.

# Eight

## VIOLENCE

I never liked the word "fight" to describe acting against an active killer because a fight typically denotes a battle between two entities with equal resources and chances to prevail. So, the *V* in ALIVE stands for violence. Although violence is typically thought of as a negative word, in this case, it may very well be the deciding factor in your survival if you're ever in a confrontation with an active killer.

Essentially, violence is another word for attack, which is what you will need to do if you're unable to leave the area or impede the active killer, and he is close enough to harm you. This may not be easy for you, but you have to understand that it is either you or the killer who is going to die. You *must* attack the killer with the intent to kill because there is no negotiating with an active killer.

### Intend to Kill
You cannot hesitate or hold back. Do not try to just maim or injure the killer, wounding them just enough to lessen the threat. The odds

are that you will fail and likely anger the killer, turning all his attention and intention to bringing you harm. And do not try to talk him or her out of killing you. Active killers are not there to vent or negotiate. They are there to kill as many people as possible in as short a time as possible—end of story!

I know that it sounds terrible to tell you to attack someone with the intent of ending that person's life, but that person wants to kill you. Active killers don't care that you just had a new baby or grand-baby, that you're a good person who always gives back to the community, or that you are a mere four days from retiring and enjoying life. *They don't care!*

All these people care about is ending your life. That's it. That's all they want. They want you dead. Gone. Existing no more.

That's why you need to be 100 percent committed to the process of taking them out. Not 80 percent or 90 percent, because whatever percentage you don't give is now on their side. Rest assured, they will use what you give them to their advantage, so don't give them anything.

Now, if you don't think you could kill someone (I get about one person in every four classes who feels this way), then change the way you look at it. Think about your family. Think about your loved ones. Could you take a life if it meant that you could go home to them? Or, if they're with you, could you take a life to make sure they survive?

I play a little game I call "Can I take another human's life?" with those few who say they cannot when I ask during my presentations. I ask the participant's name—we'll call her Mary—and then I ask Mary to mentally picture the person who means the most to her in life. It's usually a child, parent, grandparent, brother, or sister. I ask the name of that person, and then I ask for a volunteer from the audience to come up and stand next to me.

At that point, I tell Mary that the volunteer is that person she said meant the most to her. (Let's say it's her son, Jimmy.) I tell Mary to make her hand look like a gun and point it at me. I then make my hand into a gun and point it at Jimmy's head. I tell Mary, "I'm going to count to three, and when I reach three, I'm going to pull the trigger and blow Jimmy's brains all over this auditorium, and then I'm going to point the gun at you and pull the trigger. Now, Mary, tell me, could you take another human's life?" The answer has always been *yes*. I know this is a very graphic illustration, but I want to make the strongest impact possible, so class participants truly understand the point and are empowered to save their lives or those of their loved ones.

I hope you can do this. I hope you can summon the mental strength to put you and your family's needs before those of a killer. In the end, it's going to either be you or them. Only one of you is going to survive the encounter. Make sure it's you!

## Find a Weapon

If you don't regularly carry a weapon—such as a gun or a knife that you've trained with and are certified and/or capable of using (which is more than 99 percent of you, especially at work)—then now is the time to find a weapon. Arm yourself with anything you can find in your immediate vicinity to take down the attacker.

Even something as simple as a pen works. When the would-be attacker comes through the door of your office, shove it into their eyeball, driving it right into their brain. It sounds barbaric, but you need to do whatever you must do to make sure you are the one who is going home that night.

Other items that could easily serve as a weapon in an office or educational environment include a pair of scissors, a nail file, a leg broken off a table or a chair, a heavy coffee mug, or pretty much anything else you can reach that you could use against your attacker. A fire extinguisher could stand in for a weapon to spray or hit them with, as could a metal trash can, a keyboard, or most any other item you can pick up and use to strike the killer.

It doesn't matter so much what the item is; what matters is that you use it in a way that is able to stop the threat. Go for the eyes, the nose, or the throat. It doesn't matter how big the attacker is; these areas hurt when hit. Strike them with so much power that you imagine driving your weapon to the back side of the attacker's head.

Fight with the strength and tenacity you'd expect your child or your parent or your sibling to fight with if he or she were in your shoes. Use every muscle in your body, every ounce of power you have, so you're the one who can hug your loved ones another day.

Unfortunately, I've spoken with some corporate representatives about hiring me to give my presentation to their employees, but when I describe the violence portion of my course, they respond with concern because their corporate culture discourages violence, or they don't want to upset some of their staff members who might be offended by encouraging violence. Guess what, people: when that killer comes through your door with the intent of wiping out everyone in that building, it's time to throw the rainbows-and-unicorns fairyland thinking out the window and start figuring out a way to survive, which may mean taking another human's life through an act of violence.

## Swarm if You Can

If possible, swarm the killer and attack him or her as a group. While the killer may be able to overpower just one person, this becomes exponentially more difficult when faced with a whole group of people. That's why, if you can, you want to execute your violent response as a team.

To give my trainees an idea of what this looks like, I show the video of the day President Ronald Reagan was shot. Once those shots were fired, the Secret Service and other law-enforcement officials instantly swarmed John Hinckley Jr. and completely incapacitated him. (Yes, those officers were trained and retrained on how to act in such an event. And someday, probably sooner than you think, we will have the training I and others in my industry offer to employees, students, and others as a standard in workplaces, schools, hospitals, places of worship, and anywhere else people congregate.)

This is exactly what you want to do to an active killer if there is a group of you. You want to swarm him or her to gain control over the weapon, the person, and the situation to stop the threat.

If the killer has a firearm, the swarm response involves the closest and/or strongest person grabbing the muzzle of the gun or the hand holding the knife, while the rest swarm the assailant to immobilize him or her.

When seeking to gain control of the weapon, you should grab it with every ounce of strength you have. Imagine that it's your child, and someone is trying to take the child from you. Use brute force, and don't let it happen.

Since the muzzle directs where the bullet will go when fired, you must control it to dictate the direction of the bullet. That's why your goal is to keep the muzzle pointed down whenever possible; if fired, the bullet, it is hoped, would hit someone only in the leg if the person is in front of the shooter. If the action is carried out properly, the gunman can only get off one shot before the weapon is rendered inoperative.

It also helps if you're able to control the firing ability of the gun. After all, if no bullets can come out of it, then no one can be shot. While that doesn't necessarily remove all the danger in an active killer situation, it does help level the playing field between you and the killer.

One way to disable a handgun, which could be a revolver or semiautomatic with a visible hammer, is to grab the weapon so your thumb or finger is placed between the hammer and the frame of the gun, preventing the hammer from dropping if the trigger is pulled, so the firing pin doesn't contact the primer of the bullet.

You could also cause a jam by tightly gripping the frame and slide of a semiautomatic handgun so that, if the trigger is pulled, the slide would not have enough kinetic energy from the recoil to eject the spent round and rack a new one, causing a jam. (For those of you not familiar with handgun nomenclature, just grab the gun as tightly as you can, with both hands if possible, while keeping the end of the gun pointed away from you and others, and the gun will jam, making it difficult, if not impossible, to fire again.)

In the case of a would-be killer using an edged weapon or blunt object, the same principle applies. The first or most appropriate person should immediately control the weapon, while the others swarm to control the assailant.

Remember: When swarming, your first goal should be to control the weapon. Secondarily, you want to disable the killer, separating the weapon from him or her if you can.

## Size Doesn't Matter

This is the point where some people may object, saying that they're too small or too weak to take on a large attacker. However, if you've been in my classes, you've seen the video where two small females swarm a shooter as he enters the room. The first controls the gun while the second jumps on top of him. They were completely, 100 percent committed, so they took him down.

This proves that size does *not* matter. If you want to go home to your loved ones, if you have enough drive to be the one who walks away alive, you *can* achieve your goal. This is true whether you have two people to swarm the killer or twenty. Your mindset and your motivation will help you survive.

If you're ever faced with this type of situation, make a conscious decision to attack the killer with every ounce of your being, armed with the knowledge that if you do not kill them, they *will* kill you! How do you know this? Because active killers want to kill as many people as possible in as short a period as possible. History has shown that this is their primary goal.

They already know that their lives are most likely going to end, that the likelihood of them walking away from the situation alive is minimal so they have nothing to lose. This means the only way you're going to dominate them is to have a greater determination to live than they have for you to die.

# Nine

## EXPOSE

The last step to surviving an active killer incident is what I refer
to as EXPOSE. In other words, once you believe the event has
ended, it's time to evaluate your situation again, and, if you've determined that it's safe to do so, expose your position.

The key to exposing your position in a way that continues to
help you avoid harm is to do it *carefully*. There are plenty of reasons
for being so cautious when revealing where you have been during the
incident.

## Being Careful Is the Key, for Many Reasons

For starters, you can't always be sure where the bad guy is. Because sounds
tend to travel, especially down long hallways, the noises that you think
are coming from one area or location may be coming from another.

Therefore, if you decide to expose yourself and go on the move,
instead of walking *away* from danger, you may discover that you're
walking toward it. This could put you face-to-face with a killer who

wouldn't have even known you were there or had access to you if you'd just stayed in place.

Secondarily, as we've discussed in previous chapters, sometimes active killers work in pairs or teams (like the husband-and-wife team in San Bernardino or the two active shooters at Columbine). This means that although one active killer may have moved past you or may be physically down, incapacitated and unable to move, that doesn't necessarily mean that the threat is over.

There could very well be another killer somewhere else in the vicinity. Expose yourself too early, and you could find yourself hurt or killed when you wouldn't have been if, again, you had stayed in your safe area.

A third reason to be careful when exposing your position is that while *you* may know that you're not the one responsible for all the killings, law enforcement does not know. Until they've had adequate time to sort out and process the scene, which can take hours, everyone is a suspect.

This means that any sudden, unanticipated, or perceived aggressive movement on your part, or an object in your hand that could be mistaken as a weapon, is likely to provoke a response on the part of law enforcement, and at an active kill incident, their primary mission is to shoot to kill. Even the most seasoned cop in a situation like this, amped on adrenaline and surrounded by carnage, might react with aggression if faced with surprise and the perception of a threat. The cop's only goal is to stop the threat, which is why you don't want to be mistaken for that threat.

## Stay Put if You Can

Because of these types of potential issues, it's always best to stay put if you can. If you're in a secure location, wait! There is absolutely no reason to rush to get out. Yes, it's likely that you're extremely scared, and yes, you probably want to get as far away from that location as possible, but the more you move around, the more you increase the potential dangers you face.

Before choosing to expose your location, use this as another opportunity to pause and assess your situation before acting in a way that could cause you harm. Remind yourself that the killer may not be where you think or may not be working alone.

Additionally, although you know that you're an innocent victim in the attack, law-enforcement officials don't, so you don't want to add to the confusion.. The less movement the better, at least until the police issue you a directive.

## Listen to Directives

Once law enforcement is on scene and telling you to come out, exit with your hands up and palms empty! Just as your heart is racing, and your mind is on full alert due to the situation at hand, the same is true for the responding officers. So, if they see something shiny in your hand—even something innocent like a cell phone or car keys—they may mistake it for a weapon and respond accordingly.

The best way to avoid any misinterpretations of this nature is to have absolutely nothing in your hands. The less room there is for error, the more likely it is that you'll go home as quickly and as safely as possible.

Even if you had a gun or something else to protect yourself during the incident, now is the time to set it down, preferably in a location that is out of your reach. This will help make it clearer to the police that, now that they are here, you have no intention of picking the weapon up and using it. This also helps the officers know that they are safe with you, that you are *not* an active killer, which ultimately makes you safer with them.

Whatever instructions or directives the police give to you, follow them. Even if you don't understand why they're telling you to do or not do something, understand that they know more about the situation than you, and trust that whatever it is they're telling you to do is in your best interest.

And if they start to ask you questions, tell them what you know in as few words as possible. Although you'll likely want to share every little detail, partly because of the adrenaline racing through your blood and partly because it would be a huge stress relief to tell your story, it helps to realize that they only need the information that can help them determine (1) where the active killer is located, (2) whether he or she is working alone, and (3) where any potential victims are located.

Everything else at that point is secondary, so don't worry about getting it out just yet. You'll be interviewed in depth as soon as the situation is under control, and you can share it all then. But, for now, just share the information they need to know.

## Fight the Urge to Run

Again, if you're in a secure area, don't run if you think you're safe. Stay where you are until law-enforcement officials tell you that it's clear to come out. It may be tempting, and your urge to flee may be growing, especially if you've been locked in your area for an extended period, but you're safer if you're stationary, if the event has ended.

Only when you're confident that the danger is over should you expose yourself. Even then, you want to come out with your hands up and exit the area with law enforcement's permission, if possible. By following these few simple guidelines, you increase the likelihood that you'll survive an active killer incident.

## If Unsure, Contact Dispatch

If you're unsure at all about whether it's safe to expose yourself—maybe you haven't heard movement in a long time, yet police still haven't told you to come out—you can always call 911 and talk to a dispatcher. He or she can then advise you whether you should move from your location.

Ideally, you'd already contacted them when the incident began to report what was happening and so that responding law enforcement knew where you were and that you were safe. But if not, now is an appropriate time to call. They'll know what is going on and can communicate with law enforcement on the scene to give you the best advice.

Just make sure you speak quietly and continue to stay aware in case the situation truly hasn't ended. The less noise you make, the lower the chance that an active killer would be drawn to your location. Therefore, your cell phone should still be on silent as well.

Exposing your location in an active killer incident is one of the most potentially dangerous times for you, so it should always be done with care and, if possible, at a police officer's request. The other thing you can do to create a more successful response is to work as a team. We covered that briefly in the last chapter when we talked about swarming, but let's go into that more in-depth in the next chapter because, as you'll soon learn, this one principle can be critical to surviving an active killer incident.

# Ten

## Work as a Team

On March 18, 2017, *Harvard Business Review (HBR)* posted an article titled "How to Keep Your Team Focused and Productive during Uncertain Times." At the beginning of this piece, *HBR*'s contributing editor and the author of the article, Amy Gallo, says, "Whether it's political turmoil or a reorganization at your company, employees who are concerned about their future are likely to be distracted and unproductive."[48] Gallo goes on to say that this type of response "can be contagious," ultimately negatively affecting the whole team.

Unfortunately, the same issue can and does occur during an active killer incident, when innocent bystanders and victims become concerned about the fate of their own future. This results in feeling distracted and contributes to unproductive actions directed toward the situation, often inciting others around them to feel and respond the same way.

The only difference is that, instead of it's being their jobs that are at risk, it's their lives. This makes having a cohesive and effective team response critical to everyone's survival.

## The Importance of a Healthy Team Mentality

If you've ever played sports, then you already understand how team performance can impact both your individual and collective team results. Work together cohesively, and you can take yourselves and your team to the championship. Work solely as individuals, without utilizing each member's strengths and contributions, and you'll be lucky to win a game or two.

Having a team mentality in active killer incidents can greatly impact your ability to survive. It involves learning how to focus on self-preservation while still acting as a team, so you'll have a solid chance of survival.

That's why, if possible, you should all do your training together as a team. When each one of you knows exactly what to do and how to respond, it reduces the need to educate everyone about what actions you should and shouldn't take. You're able to just act with minimal communication (and minimal delay) because everyone is on the same page.

There's another benefit of practicing active killer survival as a team. When you do this, there will inevitably be fewer "low-hanging fruits."

## Active Killers and "Low-Hanging Fruit"

"Low-hanging fruit" in an active killer situation refers to the individuals who are the easiest to reach, thus the easiest to kill. This includes the people who don't know how or where to best hide, how to lock and block the door to impede, and all the other principles you've already learned in this book and/or my course.

Because the active killer's goal is to take as many lives as possible in as short a time as possible, these types of people are preferred, largely because they offer the active killer the opportunity to get the most kills. They make his or her mission much easier.

Knowing this, if you ever find yourself in an active killer event, you must focus on the people in your immediate vicinity who are the easiest targets, the low-hanging fruit. It's also your responsibility to not fall into that category and, if possible, to help others avoid that label as well.

## Train as a Team

Everyone should have the same training, so that each one of you is intimately familiar with the same effective active killer survival response. Everyone must learn and practice ALIVE *the same way*, executing their response as a team!

Remember, in times of stress, your body and mind will default, or revert, to your training. Your body and mind will subconsciously know what to do and will help you do it, even if you learned the initial skills quite a while ago. Train as a team, then, and you'll increase the likelihood that you'll work together like a well-oiled machine.

This training enables you to respond quickly and more effectively because you will all know what to do. It's like having a team of mechanics working on a race car or a team of doctors working on a surgery. When each one can do his or her own part, and everyone else involved knows it, that makes everyone's chances of (and confidence in) success that much greater.

## Perform Active Killer Drills

One way to accomplish this type of teamwork is to regularly perform active killer drills in your workplace, hospital, school, or house of worship. Whether you're the employer or the supervisor in charge, the administrator, the principal, or the head of the church, making these drills mandatory on a quarterly or semiannual basis could be the difference between having a building full of people who are able to successfully defend themselves against an active killer or having to tell their family members that your negligence left them unprepared.

This may sound harsh, but it's a sad reality because that's exactly what you'll be doing if you don't train your staff in active killer response, and an incident occurs. It's also one that isn't new because drills have been used for ages to help create a more effective response.

Take schools and fire drills, for instance. The National Fire Protection Association recommends that schools conduct fire drills every thirty days, at a minimum, during the school year.[49] Why is this so important? To keep fires like the one that happened more than half a century ago (which killed ninety students) from ever happening again.

## Lessons Learned from Fire

In the 1950s, schools didn't practice fire prevention by way of fire drills like they do today. So, when a fire started at roughly 2:30 p.m. on December 1, 1958, at Our Lady of Angels School in Chicago, Illinois, neither students nor teachers were prepared to respond.

This resulted in widespread panic, causing some students to jump from the second floor (whether there was someone there to catch them or not) and causing others to remain right where they were, simply "praying for help."[50] By the time all was said and done, ninety students—which was almost one-tenth of the total student body— had lost their lives, as had three nuns.

Now schools make it a priority to practice an effective response in the event of a fire starting during the school day. This only makes sense because it *does* happen, quite regularly, in fact; statistics provided by the Federal Emergency Management Agency (FEMA) indicate that school fires occur at the rate of four thousand per year in the

United States alone.[51] Because of nationwide, mandatory fire drills in schools, not a single student has died in a school fire in over fifty years.

Doesn't it make sense, then, to practice active killer drills? These incidents are happening regularly too, so why leave your response up to chance? Plan for these types of incidents, and plan for them as a team, much the same way that you do for earthquakes, tornadoes, nuclear blasts, and any other type of disaster that serves as a possible threat to the safety of you and your staff. The difference is that whereas many of those types of events occur regionally, active shooter events can happen anywhere and anytime.

## Active Killer Response Advances

Fortunately, we are seeing some advances in this arena already, such as the audible alerts, cell-phone apps, or mass texts that are issued, warning everyone in the area that there is an active shooter situation. This helps initiate a team response more quickly and effectively, giving everyone in the vicinity a better chance of survival until the threat can be stopped. And as stated earlier, some law-enforcement agencies now utilize text-to-911, so an emergency can be reported via text in the event the reporting party cannot call.

It's also now possible for businesses to purchase products that could prove to be invaluable in an active killer situation. This includes the following items:

- First-aid and trauma kits
- Tourniquets and other bleeding controls
- Door blocks and locks
- Window covers
- Camera-based security systems

- And, of course, the most effective but arguably the most controversial tool in a school or workplace: an actual weapon. (More and more schools, medical facilities, and workplaces are beginning to approve the carrying of weapons by qualified, authorized people.)

By having these things in place at your business, school, or other places you frequent, you can more effectively plan, prepare for, and respond to an active killer incident. Use these items in your regular drills so you know exactly how to utilize them in the event of an actual incident.

At the end of this book, there are some practical exercises that you can use to get started when creating your drills. Use them, or feel free to create your own. Ideally, you want to plan for as many different situations as possible, so you'll be more prepared should an active killer ever decide to strike where you are located. You can *never* be too prepared for a situation like this, so practice your responses regularly and consistently. This practice may just save your life and the lives of those around you.

# Conclusion

Surviving an active killer incident is never a guarantee. There's no one thing you can do that will 100 percent ensure that you will make it through an incident alive. However, there are many things you can do that will improve your odds dramatically, and we've covered several of them in this book.

What can you do to stay ALIVE? Let's do a quick recap.

**Assess.** The first thing you want to do in an active killer incident is assess your situation. This involves processing what's happening around you and using that information to determine your next steps. It means asking yourself questions like these:
- Where is the killer?
- Where are the exits?
- Can I run?
- If you can't run, can you impede the killer or safely hide?
- If you can't impede, what can you use to fight?

During this assessment, you must also mentally prepare yourself to kill or be killed. Remember that it's either you or the killer going home tonight. Make a commitment that it will be you.

While it's normal to freeze for a second or two, train yourself regularly so that you aren't left sitting there like a deer in the headlights.

**Leave.** If possible, the best action you can take is to leave the scene. Get as far away as possible, so you're not close enough to be killed or injured.

Notify others while you go. If you have a PA system or an app that is available to notify people near the event, use it. The more innocent bystanders you can get away from the area, the more lives that will likely be saved.

Also, when leaving, use a command presence. Don't be afraid to take charge of the situation and the people in it. Talk to those around you with authority, so they'll be willing to leave the area safely with you. Get as far away from the threat as possible as quickly as possible, and direct others to follow you.

If you can't get out of the building, at least get safely to a secure location within that facility. Ideally, this would be a safe room with no windows, a reinforced front, and camera intercoms so insiders can see who is outside the room.

If the people with you have been through this training, they'll know where this is and will go there automatically. If not, then it may take some direction on your part to help those around you pick a safe place to wait out the event.

When you go, take only your cell phone and weapon, if you have one. More and more states are actively issuing concealed firearms licenses, so people carry guns. If you have one, and your place of employment allows you to have it, take it to your safe room, keeping it hidden unless and until you're ready to use it.

**Impede.** Once you're in a safe area, impede the killer's opportunity and ability to get to you. One way to do this is to lock and block (lock the door and block it with as many things as possible, with the heaviest items closest to the door).

Your goal at this point is to become as invisible as possible by making it appear that no one is present in the room. You can do this by hiding behind objects. (Remember the principle of cover versus concealment; your best place to hide is behind something that will stop a bullet.) Additionally, cover any windows to the room so you cannot be seen.

Effectively impeding an attacker occurs when you make yourself a "hard target." The more difficulties the killer has in reaching you, the more likely it is that he or she will pass by you.

**Violence.** While locked and blocked in your safe area, arm yourself with anything you can find to injure or disable the attacker in the event he or she gains entry to the room. Understand that it is you or him, so you must attack the killer with the intent to kill!

If you have people with you and it's at all possible, swarm the attacker. Attack him or her as a group, control the weapon (muzzle down and keep it from firing, if you can), and disable the killer so he or she can do no further harm.

**Expose.** If you are in a secure location, stay there until directed otherwise by law enforcement. If you must leave, once you believe the event has ended, it's time to evaluate your situation and expose your position carefully.

Because there may be additional attackers, you don't want to give your location away too soon. Plus, law enforcement won't know that you're not a bad guy, so follow all their commands as precisely as possible. This will help keep you safe until the event is over, everything is sorted out, and you can return home to your loved ones.

## Be a Sheepdog

As I stated in my introduction, in Lt. Col. Dave Grossman's book, *On Combat, The Psychology and Physiology of Deadly Conflict in War and in Peace*, he writes, "Most of the people in our society are sheep. They are kind, gentle, productive creatures who can only hurt one another by accident." Grossman also goes on to explain, "Then there are the wolves and the wolves feed on the sheep without mercy…Then there are the sheepdogs and I am a sheepdog. I live to protect the flock and confront the wolf. [52]"

Remember, if you have no capacity for violence, then you are a healthy, productive citizen. You are a sheep. On the other hand, if you have a capacity for violence and no empathy for your fellow citizens, then you can be defined as an aggressive sociopath. A wolf.

But what if you have a capacity for violence and a deep love for your fellow citizens?

In this case, you are a sheepdog. A warrior. Someone who is walking the hero's path. Someone who can walk into the heart of darkness, into the universal human phobia, and walk out unscathed. Someone who can live through an active killer attack.

## The World Is Changing

The world is constantly changing. While some of these changes are undeniably good, some are not. One that is not is that evil people are committing more and more evil acts, making such incidents more common now than ever before.

Sadly, this situation is not likely to get better in our lifetime either. With the growth of radical terror-based groups like ISIS, we will undoubtedly find more and more wolves in our society. More and more people intent on doing us harm in larger-scale attacks.

This means that we need to develop a zero-tolerance policy, one in which situations like these are not tolerated by the masses. A standard must be established so the perpetrators of evil know they and their actions will not be tolerated. That they will not make victims of us; we will make victims of them. Many people are fighting hard to take us in that direction, me included, but we're not there yet. And we likely won't be there anytime soon.

That's why you must be as prepared as possible by adopting survival and security mindsets and practicing proactive reactionism. Instead of being on the defense by way of reaction, you must be prepared to be on the offense. You need to be diligent in your trainings by performing practical exercises and drills (like the ones at the end of this book), so that you know exactly how to respond when needed.

**You need to be a sheepdog. You need to stay ALIVE!**

# Implementing ALIVE: Practical Exercises

This section includes many scenarios for you and your team to think about, plan for, and practice when using the ALIVE active killer response plan that you've just learned. As you go through each one, remember to do the following things:

- **Assess.** Stop, breathe, process what's happening, and consider your next steps. Ask yourself: Where is the killer? Where are the exits? Can you run? If you can't run, can you impede? If you can't impede, what can you use to fight? Mentally prepare yourself to kill or be killed, and be prepared to act!

- **Leave.** If you can exit the building, run as far away as possible. Also, tell everyone within earshot what you believe is happening, if possible, using a command presence to get them to leave too. Leave all your belongings behind but your cell phone (which you should be on, calling 911) and a weapon, if you have one. Run in the opposite direction of the threat if that's where the most accessible exit is. The alternative is to run to a secure location (a safe room) if that is closer.

- **Impede.** Practice a lock-and-block response. Shut and lock the door if possible. If the door doesn't have a lock on it, come up with other ways to make it harder to open. Cover the windows and switch your cell phones to silent. Secure the door from entry by placing the heaviest items in the room against it first. Find a place to hide, preferably one that provides cover in addition to concealment.

- **Violence.** Prepare for the killer's entry. Control the weapon (muzzle down) and, if possible, inhibit its firing ability. Use your own weapon. Is swarming an option? Everyone stay on top of the attacker, and call dispatch or yell to law enforcement advising them where you are. Bottom line: attack with the intent to kill!

- **Expose.** If you are in a secure location, *wait*! Is the event over? Is there more than one shooter or killer? Have you received instructions from law enforcement? Are you on the phone with support, such as 911 dispatch? When you finally decide to exit, exit with your hands up and empty! Follow their instructions, and tell them what you know in as few words as possible.

Also, once you've trained with a scenario, change up some of the facts to practice different responses. This will not only better prepare you but also train your mind to consider the fact that there are many ways a scenario can go. This will help keep you more alert, so you can respond to the situation faster and more effectively as it unfolds.

For instance, if you imagined one active killer, try going through the scenario and imagining two or three. Or, if you could impede, and the active killer walked by in the first scenario, practice the same scenario with the active killer attempting to breach the door. Then practice it again with him or her gaining entry. The more scenarios you're prepared for, the more prepared you'll be in the event of an active killer incident.

Finally, train as individuals *and* as teams. When training in teams, think about who would be best suited for what type of response. For example, if you're impeding the active killer, are some team members more capable of moving the heavier items against the door? Or, if the killer gains entry, who is going to attempt to secure the muzzle while everyone else swarms? Practice with each team member playing different roles in the scenarios so each person is more familiar and comfortable with each one.

## Scenarios to Practice

Now that you're ready to implement the ALIVE active killer response, here are some scenarios to consider:

- You're working at your desk and hear gunfire by the front door and people screaming. What do you do?
- You're at work, standing by the front desk talking to a co-worker, when a former employee walks in with a long gun. What do you do?
- You're at the grocery store with your family, about ready to check out, and see a man with a gun enter the store. What do you do?
- You're at your place of worship and, in the middle of the service, someone comes in through the rear door with a gun. What do you do?
- You're in line at your favorite fast-food place in the food court at the local mall, and you see a gunman walking down the corridor, coming toward you. What do you do?
- You're at a parade and see a man with what appears to be explosive devices strapped to his chest walk up and stand just a few feet away. What do you do?
- You're at a concert and see a man in front of you begin to stab other concertgoers while shouting. What do you do?
- You're at the airport, ready to go on a nice, relaxing vacation, when you see someone attack a police officer with a long-bladed knife. What do you do?
- You're out to eat and about to dive into your dinner when someone walks in and starts shooting. What do you do?
- You're at the movies with friends and, in the middle of the movie, you notice someone walk in the side door with a gun. What do you do?

- You're at the bar for an after-work drink, and someone walks in with a machete. You're sitting right by the door. What do you do?
- You're waiting in your vehicle to pick your kids up from school and notice a man with a rifle walking toward the school. What do you do?

I hope none of these scenarios will *ever* happen to you. However, if they do, at least you'll be prepared to deal with them as effectively as possible. At least you will have given yourself a chance to walk away ALIVE!

# Afterward

A couple of weeks after the Route 91 Harvest Music Festival shooting in Las Vegas, I received an e-mail that made the thousands of hours I've spent creating, updating, and teaching my ALIVE active shooter survival training worth every minute of effort.

Mr. Julian,

My name is Liz Moreno. I worked for about six years at a place called International Immunology in Murrieta, California, where you came in and gave us your active shooter survival training course. It was interesting, very informative, and I enjoyed it but never in a million years thought that I'd have to use it.

On October 1, I was in Las Vegas at the Route 91 Harvest Festival, standing at the right of the stage with my boyfriend watching Jason Aldean perform. Suddenly there was a sound like firecrackers coming from the right of us. Jason and the band ran off the stage. We turned around and two people were shot behind us, one in the face and one in the chest. Everyone immediately went forward and got down on the ground in a big pile. Right then, in that very moment when the third round of shots went off, as I was lying there attempting to cover my neck and head with my arm, your training that I had listened to years prior instantly popped into my head. I told my boyfriend, "We need to run. We cannot stay here! When he stops to reload next time, I am running!" He was hesitant at first, but I think he could tell that I was running either way. He grabbed my hand, and we ran as fast as we could, staying low and stopping to hide while shots were fired, then sprinting again in between. We ran straight to the

Excalibur, where we were staying, and I sent a text to my parents at 10:14 p.m. from the lobby of Excalibur. That is how quickly we were out of there.

I truly believe taking your training is what told me to make that decision and say without a doubt that we have to run, which ultimately saved us. Had we stayed there we may have gotten shot; had we hesitated longer we could have been trampled or who knows what.

I know I'm just one of many that have had your training course, but I just wanted to let you know that I truly believe in that split second it saved our lives.

Thank you,
Liz Moreno

I met with Liz and her boyfriend shortly after receiving her letter, and we talked about her experience. She became very emotional while reliving this terrifying event, but I needed to know exactly how the training helped her, so I could build on that in future trainings.

What Liz told me emphatically fueled my desire to teach as many people the ALIVE program as quickly as I could. Liz stated that she hadn't thought about the training since attending my class three years ago, but, in that moment, when she thought to herself, "This could be it; I could die today," the training came rushing back to her like a slap in the face, and she knew exactly what she needed to do. So, she ran, taking cover when the firing started again and running when it stopped.

As I stated in chapter 4, people default to their level of training and remember years later how to perform CPR or the Heimlich maneuver. In this instance, that training helped save Liz and her boyfriend's lives, but unfortunately for many who never had a chance, some stayed to wait out the gunfire but never made it home.

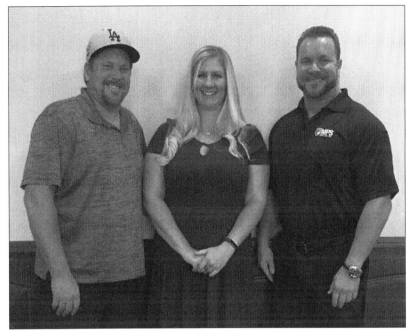

*Liz Moreno and her boyfriend, Martin Bangma* (left), *when they visited me at my corporate headquarters in Southern California.*

# In Memoriam

I wanted to provide photographs for several active shooter events, but rather than spotlighting the killers by showing pictures of them (further perpetuating their memory, which is exactly what they would want and which therefore I refuse to do), I've included photos of the victims and the loving memorials created in their memory. These are the people whose faces should be etched in our memories, not the culprits of these unforgivable acts.

This list is certainly not comprehensive, and because of a lack of data available during my research, unfortunately I am unable to present more photos of the fallen. Those not shown in these pages should be remembered just as vividly as those who are shown.

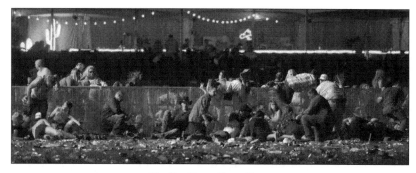

*Credit: Getty Contributor*

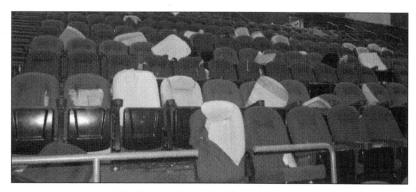

*Credit: Aurora, CO, Police Department*

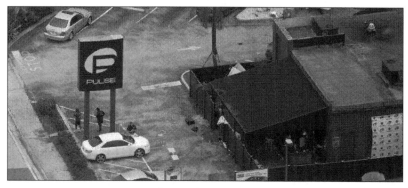

*Credit: Carlo Allegri/Reuters*

On April 20, 1999, two teens, Eric Harris, eighteen, and Dylan Klebold, seventeen, went on a shooting spree at Columbine High School in Littleton, Colorado, killing thirteen people and wounding more than twenty others before turning their guns on themselves. This was the worst high-school shooting in US history. There was speculation that the two committed the killings because they had been bullied, were members of a group of social outcasts that was fascinated by Goth culture, or had been influenced by violent video games and music.

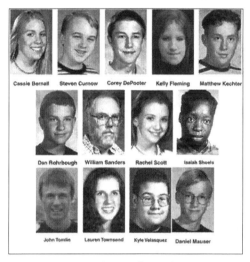

*Credit: Daily Mail*

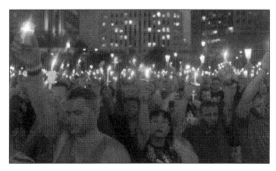

*Credit: Drew Angerer/Getty Images*

A series of coordinated shootings occurred during three weeks in October 2002 in Maryland, Virginia, and the District of Columbia. Ten people were killed, and three others were critically injured in the Washington, DC, metropolitan area and along Interstate 95 in Virginia. The shooters were John Allen Muhammad, forty-one, and Lee Boyd Malvo, seventeen.

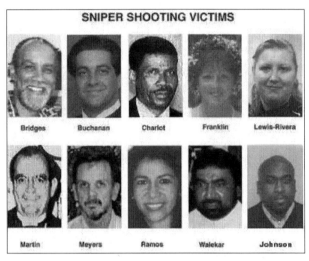

*Credit: Criminal Minds Wiki*

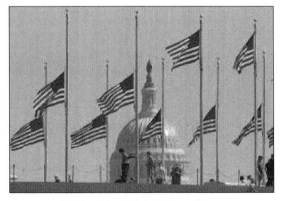

*Credit: Mark Wilson/Getty Images*

On April 16, 2007, at 7:15 a.m., Seung Hui Cho, twenty-three, armed with two handguns, began shooting in a dormitory at Virginia Polytechnic Institute and State University in Blacksburg, Virginia. Two and a half hours later, he chained the doors shut in a classroom building and began shooting at the students and faculty inside. Thirty-two people were killed; seventeen were wounded. The shooter committed suicide as police entered the building.

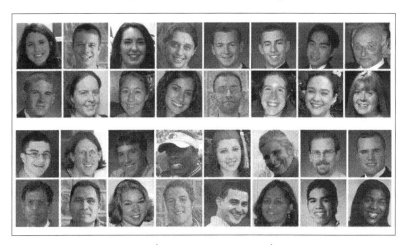

*Credit: WSET/Virginia Tech*

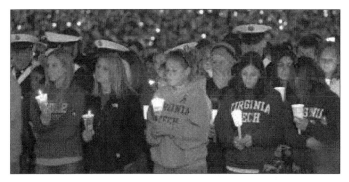

*Credit: UPI/Roger L. Wollenberg*

On November 5, 2009, at 1:20 p.m., Nidal Malik Hasan, thirty-nine, armed with two handguns, began shooting inside the Fort Hood Soldier Readiness Processing Center in Fort Hood, Texas. Thirteen people were killed; thirty-two were wounded, including one police officer. During an exchange of gunfire, the shooter was wounded and taken into custody.

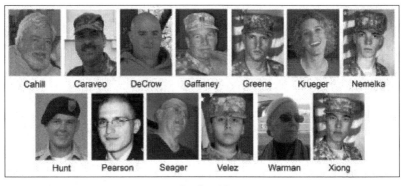

*Credit: AP*

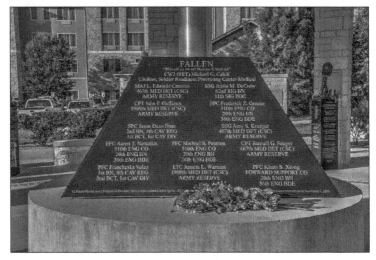

*Credit: Wikipedia*

On July 22, 2011, Anders Behring Breivik killed 8 people and injured at least 209 more using a car bomb of mixed fertilizer and fuel oil at the executive government quarter in Oslo, Norway, before opening fire at a summer camp two hours later on Utøya, an island in Tyrifjorden, killing 69 and wounding 110.

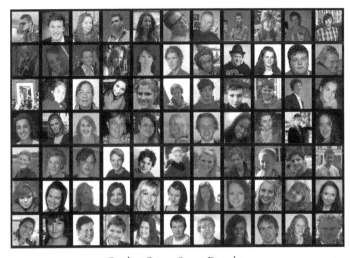

*Credit: Crime Scene Database*

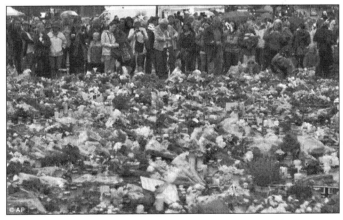

*Credit: AP*

On July 20, 2012, at 12:30 a.m., James Eagan Holmes, twenty-four, armed with a rifle, a shotgun, and a handgun, began shooting after releasing teargas canisters in a theater at the Cinemark Century 16 movie theaters in Aurora, Colorado. Twelve people were killed; fifty-eight were wounded.

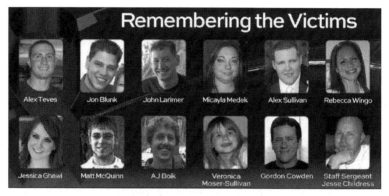

*Credit: Blogspot.com; Indy Democrat Blog*

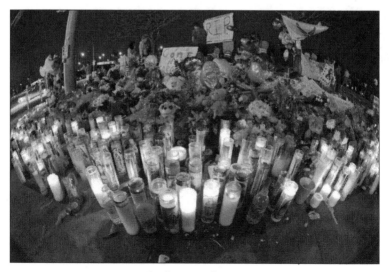

*Credit: David Harpe*

On May 23, 2014, at 9:27 p.m., Elliot Rodger, twenty-two, armed with a handgun and several knives, began shooting in the first of seventeen locations in Isla Vista, California. After stabbing three inside his apartment earlier that day, the shooter began driving through town, shooting from his car. He killed three and wounded seven, and he struck and wounded another seven with his vehicle. A total of six people were killed; fourteen were wounded. The shooter committed suicide after being wounded during an exchange of gunfire with law enforcement.

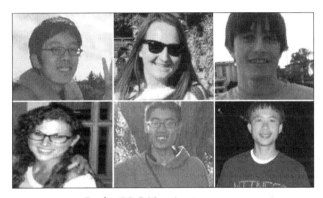

*Credit: BBC News/various sources*

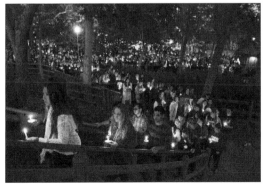

*Credit: Jae C. Hong/AP*

On December 14, 2012, at 9:30 a.m., Adam Lanza, twenty, armed with two handguns and a rifle, shot through the secured front door to enter Sandy Hook Elementary School in Newtown, Connecticut. He killed twenty students and six adults, and he wounded two adults inside the school. Prior to the shooting, the shooter killed his mother at their home. In total, twenty-seven people were killed; two were wounded. The shooter committed suicide after police arrived.

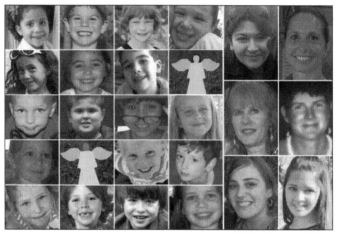

*Credit: Time (Reuters/Rex USA)*

| | |
|---|---|
| CHARLOTTE BACON, AGE 6 | GRACE MCDONNELL, AGE 7 |
| DANIEL BARDEN, AGE 7 | ANNE MARIE MURPHY, AGE 52 |
| RACHEL DAVINO, AGE 29 | EMILIE PARKER, AGE 6 |
| OLIVIA ENGEL, AGE 6 | JACK PINTO, AGE 6 |
| JOSEPHINE GAY, AGE 7 | NOAH POZNER, AGE 6 |
| ANA M. MARQUEZ-GREENE, AGE 6 | CAROLINE PREVIDI, AGE 6 |
| DYLAN HOCKLEY, AGE 6 | JESSICA REKOS, AGE 6 |
| DAWN HOCHSPRUNG, AGE 47 | AVIELLE RICHMAN, AGE 6 |
| MADELEINE HSU, AGE 6 | LAUREN ROUSSEAU, AGE 30 |
| CATHERINE HUBBARD, AGE 6 | MARY SHERLACH, AGE 56 |
| CHASE KOWALSKI, AGE 7 | VICTORIA SOTO, AGE 27 |
| JESSE LEWIS, AGE 6 | BENJAMIN WHEELER, AGE 6 |
| JAMES MATTIOLI , AGE 6 | ALLISON N. WYATT, AGE 6 |

*Credit: CBS8*

On September 16, 2013, a lone gunman, thirty-four-year-old Aaron Alexis, fatally shot twelve people and injured three others in a mass shooting at the headquarters of the Naval Sea Systems Command inside the Washington Navy Yard in southeast Washington, DC. The attack, which took place in the Navy Yard's Building 197, began around 8:16 a.m. and ended when Alexis was killed by police around 9:25 a.m.

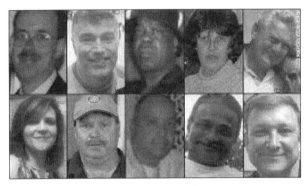

*Credit: CNN Compilation*

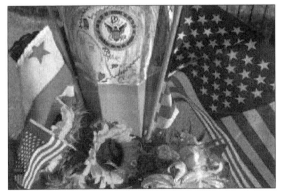

*Credit: Matt McClain/Washington Post*

On June 17, 2015, at 9:00 p.m., Dylann Storm Roof, twenty-one, armed with a rifle, began shooting at a prayer service at the Emanuel African Methodist Episcopal Church in Charleston, South Carolina. Nine people were killed; no one was wounded.

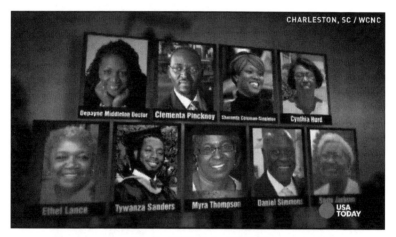

*Credit: USA Today/WCNC*

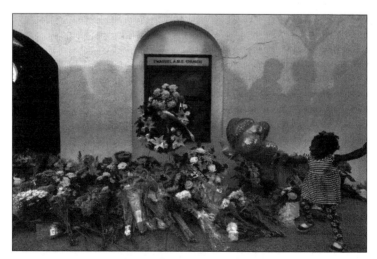

*Credit: Stephen B. Morton/AP Photo*

On July 16, 2015, at 10:51 a.m., Mohammad Youssuf Abdulazeez, twenty-four, armed with a rifle, began shooting at the Armed Forces Career Center in Chattanooga, Tennessee, wounding a US Marine. The shooter then drove to the Navy and Marine Reserve Center, where he killed four US Marines and wounded a law-enforcement officer and, a US Navy sailor who died a few days later. A total of five were killed; two were wounded, including the law-enforcement officer. The shooter was killed during an exchange of gunfire with law enforcement.

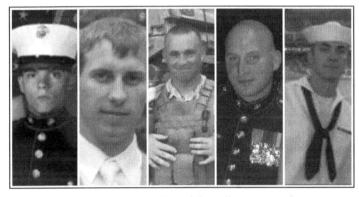

*Credit: Families of the Fallen Five*

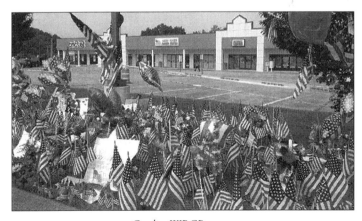

*Credit: WRCBtv.com*

On December 2, 2015, at 11:30 a.m., husband and wife Syed Rizwan Farook, twenty-eight, and Tashfeen Malik, twenty-nine, armed with two rifles, two handguns, and an explosive device, began shooting in the parking lot of the Inland Regional Center in San Bernardino, California. They moved inside the building, shooting at coworkers of one of the shooters. Fourteen people were killed; twenty-two were wounded. The shooters fled the scene; they were killed a few hours later during an exchange of gunfire with law enforcement.

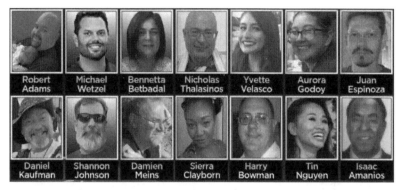

*Credit: CNN*

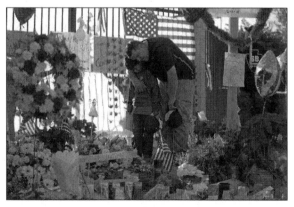

*Credit: AP*

On June 12, 2016, at approximately 2:00 a.m., Omar Mateen, twenty-nine, armed with an assault rifle and one pistol, began shooting inside the Pulse nightclub, a dance club in Orlando, Florida. After an extended period during which the shooter barricaded himself, police entered the club and killed the shooter. Forty-nine people were killed; fifty-three were wounded.

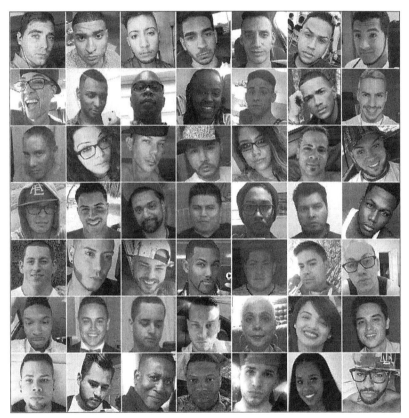

*Credit: DailyMail.co.uk*

On October 1, 2017, Stephen Paddock opened fire on the audience of the Route 91 Harvest Country Music Festival from the thirty-second floor of the Mandalay Bay Hotel and Casino in Las Vegas, Nevada, killing fifty-eight people and wounding over five hundred before killing himself just before law enforcement breached the room.

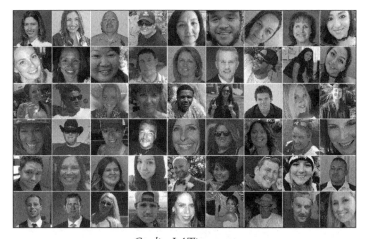

*Credit: LATimes.com*

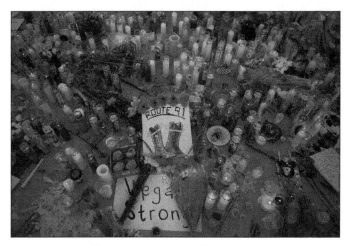

*Credit: Drew Angerer/Getty Images*

On November 5, 2017, a mass shooting occurred at the First Baptist Church in Sutherland Springs, Texas, about thirty miles east of the city of San Antonio. The gunman was twenty-six-year-old Devin Patrick Kelley of nearby New Braunfels, who killed twenty-six people and injured twenty others. He was shot twice by a male civilian as he exited the church. Fleeing in his SUV, Kelley crashed after a high-speed chase and was found dead with multiple gunshot wounds, including a self-inflicted shot to the head.

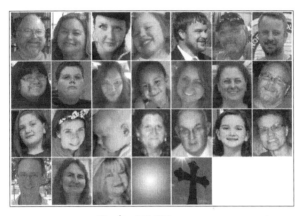

*Credit: NBCNews.com*

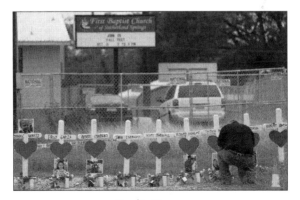

*Credit: Reuters*

# 2000–2016 Active Shooter Incidents Ending in Suicide

Below is a list of active shooter incidents identified by the FBI in the United States in which the killer committed suicide. The methodology to include or exclude an incident on this list was established and articulated in the FBI's study of active shooter events released in 2014. See J. Pete Blair and Katherine W. Schweit, *A Study of Active Shooter Incidents, 2000–2013* (Washington, DC: Texas State University and Federal Bureau of Investigation, US Department of Justice, 2014).

This list is included to provide evidence of killers' predilection for ending their own lives rather than having their lives taken, at which point they would lose the sense of power and control they finally feel they have reclaimed from society and from those they believe bullied or victimized them, or otherwise deprived them of the respect they felt they deserved.

## 2001
## Amko Trading Store (Commerce)

On January 9, 2001, at 12:00 p.m., Ki Yung Park, fifty-four, fatally shot his estranged wife at a convenience store they owned in Houston, Texas. Armed with two handguns, he then drove to the nearby Amko Trading Store and continued shooting. Four people were killed; no one was wounded. The shooter committed suicide when police arrived after being flagged down by a citizen.

## Navistar International Corporation Factory (Commerce)

On February 5, 2001, at 9:40 a.m., William Daniel Baker, fifty-seven, armed with two rifles, a handgun, and a shotgun, began shooting coworkers in the Navistar International Corporation factory in Melrose Park, Illinois. He was supposed to report to prison the next day for stealing from Navistar. Four people were killed; four were wounded. The shooter committed suicide before police arrived.

## Nu-Wood Decorative Millwork Plant, Goshen, Indiana (Commerce)

On December 6, 2001, at 2:31 p.m., Robert L. Wissman, thirty-six, armed with a shotgun, began shooting in the Nu-Wood Decorative Millwork plant in Goshen, Indiana. He had been fired from his job that morning and returned in the afternoon to begin shooting. One person was killed; six were wounded. The shooter committed suicide before police arrived.

# 2002
## Bertrand Products, Inc. (Commerce)

On March 22, 2002, at 8:15 a.m., William Lockey, fifty-four, armed with a rifle and a shotgun, began shooting coworkers in the Bertrand Products, Inc., facility in South Bend, Indiana. As he attempted to flee the scene in a stolen company van, he exchanged gunfire with police, eventually committing suicide. Four people were killed; five were wounded, including three police officers.

# 2003
## Red Lion Junior High School (Education)

On April 24, 2003, at 7:34 a.m., James Sheets, fourteen, armed with three handguns, shot and killed the school principal in the cafeteria at Red Lion Junior High School in Red Lion, Pennsylvania. Though others were present at the scene, the shooter committed suicide when police arrived.

## Modine Manufacturing Company (Commerce)

On July 1, 2003, at 10:28 p.m., Jonathon W. Russell, twenty-five, armed with a handgun, began shooting coworkers in the Modine Manufacturing Company building in Jefferson City, Missouri. Three people were killed; five were wounded. The shooter fled the premises and then committed suicide during an exchange of gunfire with police.

## Lockheed Martin Subassembly Plant (Commerce)

On July 8, 2003, at 9:30 a.m., Douglas Paul Williams, forty-eight, armed with a shotgun and a rifle, began shooting in the Lockheed Martin subassembly plant in Meridian, Mississippi. Six people were killed; eight were wounded. The shooter committed suicide before police arrived.

## Andover Industries (Commerce)

On August 19, 2003, at 8:20 a.m., Richard Wayne Shadle, thirty-two, armed with four handguns, began shooting in the Andover Industries facility in Andover, Ohio, after his boss threatened to fire him. One person was killed; two were wounded. The shooter committed suicide before police arrived.

## 2004
## ConAgra Plant (Commerce)

On July 2, 2004, at 5:00 p.m., Elijah J. Brown, twenty-one, armed with a handgun, began shooting employees in the ConAgra plant in

Kansas City, Kansas. He had been laid off due to a production slow-down but was rehired six weeks prior to the incident. Six people were killed; two were wounded. The shooter committed suicide before police arrived.

## Radio Shack, Gateway Mall (Commerce)

On November 18, 2004, at 6:45 p.m., Justin Michael Cudar, twenty-five, armed with a handgun, began shooting in the Radio Shack at the Gateway Mall in Saint Petersburg, Florida. Two were killed; one was wounded. The shooter committed suicide before police arrived.

# 2005
## DaimlerChrysler's Toledo North Assembly Plant (Commerce)

On January 26, 2005, at 8:34 p.m., Myles Wesley Meyers, fifty-four, armed with a shotgun, returned from his lunch break and began shooting in DaimlerChrysler's Toledo North Assembly plant in Toledo, Ohio. He took a woman hostage before beginning to shoot at his coworkers. One person was killed; two were wounded. The shooter committed suicide before police arrived.

## Living Church of God (House of Worship)

On March 12, 2005, at 12:51 p.m., Terry M. Ratzmann, forty-four, armed with a handgun, began shooting during a Living Church of God service at the Sheraton Hotel in Brookfield, Wisconsin. Seven people were killed; four were wounded. The shooter committed suicide before police arrived.

## Red Lake High School and Residence (Education)

On March 21, 2005, at 2:49 p.m., Jeffery James Weise, sixteen, armed with a shotgun and two handguns, began shooting at Red Lake High School in Red Lake, Minnesota. Before the incident at the school, the shooter fatally shot his grandfather, who was a police officer, and another individual at their home. He then took his grandfather's police equipment, including guns and body armor, to the school. A total of nine people were killed, including an unarmed security guard, a teacher, and five students; six students were wounded. The shooter committed suicide during an exchange of gunfire with police.

## Parking Lots, Philadelphia, Pennsylvania (Open Space)

On October 7, 2005, at 10:13 a.m., Alexander Elkin, forty-five, armed with a handgun, shot two people in different parking lots in Philadelphia, Pennsylvania. He shot his ex-wife and then drove with her body in the car to kill her friend at another location. An off-duty police officer witnessed the shooting and flagged down an on-duty police officer to pursue the shooter. After an exchange of gunfire with police, the shooter retreated to his car, where he committed suicide. Two people were killed; no one was wounded.

# 2006
## Santa Barbara US Postal Processing and Distribution Center (Government/Commerce)

On January 30, 2006, at 7:15 p.m., former postal worker Jennifer San Marco, forty-four, armed with a handgun, began shooting at her previous place of employment, the Santa Barbara US Postal Processing and Distribution Center in Goleta, California. Six people were killed; no one was wounded. The shooter committed suicide before police arrived.

## Residence, Capitol Hill Neighborhood, Seattle, Washington (Residence)

On March 25, 2006, at 7:03 a.m., Kyle Aaron Huff, twenty-eight, armed with a handgun, a shotgun, and a rifle, began shooting at a rave after-party in the Capitol Hill neighborhood of Seattle, Washington. Six people were killed; two were wounded. The shooter committed suicide as police confronted him.

## Essex Elementary School and Two Residences (Education)

On August 24, 2006, at 1:55 p.m., Christopher Williams, twenty-six, armed with a handgun, shot at various locations in Essex, Vermont. He began by fatally shooting his ex-girlfriend's mother at her home and then drove to Essex Elementary School, where his ex-girlfriend was a teacher. He did not find her, but as he searched, he killed one teacher and wounded another. He then fled to a friend's home, where he wounded one person. A total of two people were killed; two were wounded. The shooter also attempted suicide by shooting himself twice but survived and was apprehended when police arrived at the scene.

## West Nickel Mines School (Education)

On October 2, 2006, at 10:30 a.m., Charles Carl Roberts IV, thirty-two, armed with a rifle, a shotgun, and a handgun, began shooting at the West Nickel Mines School in Bart Township, Pennsylvania. After the shooter entered the building, he ordered all males and adults out of the room. After a twenty-minute standoff, he began firing. The shooter committed suicide as the police began to breach the school through a window. Five people were killed; five were wounded.

# 2007
## ZigZag Net, Inc. (Commerce)
On February 12, 2007, at 8:00 p.m., Vincent Dortch, forty-four, armed with a rifle and a handgun, began shooting during a ZigZag Net, Inc., board meeting at the Naval Business Center in Philadelphia, Pennsylvania. The shooter had scheduled the board meeting to discuss a financial dispute with other board members. Three people were killed; one was wounded. The shooter committed suicide after firing at the police.

## Kenyon Press (Commerce)
On March 5, 2007, at 9:00 a.m., Alonso Jose Mendez, sixty-eight, armed with a handgun, began shooting at his coworkers in the Kenyon Press facility in Signal Hill, California. No one was killed; three were wounded. The shooter committed suicide before police arrived.

## Virginia Polytechnic Institute and State University (Education)
On April 16, 2007, at 7:15 a.m., Seung Hui Cho, twenty-three, armed with two handguns, began shooting in a dormitory at Virginia Polytechnic Institute and State University in Blacksburg, Virginia. Two and a half hours later, he chained the doors shut in a classroom building and began shooting at the students and faculty inside.

Thirty-two people were killed; seventeen were wounded. In addition, six students were injured jumping from a second-floor classroom and were not included in other reported injury totals. The shooter committed suicide as police entered the building.

## Residence, Latah County Courthouse, and First Presbyterian Church (Residence/Government/House of Worship)

On May 19, 2007, around 11:00 p.m., Jason Kenneth Hamilton, thirty-six, armed with two rifles, began shooting outside the Latah County Courthouse in Moscow, Idaho, killing one police officer and wounding two people, including another police officer. He then fled to the First Presbyterian Church across the street and continued shooting, killing a citizen and wounding two people, including another police officer. Before driving to the courthouse, he fatally shot his wife in their residence. A total of three people were killed; three were wounded. The shooter committed suicide after police arrived.

## Residence in Crandon, Wisconsin (Residence)

On October 7, 2007, at 2:45 a.m., Tyler Peterson, twenty, a sheriff's deputy armed with a rifle, began shooting during a party at his ex-girlfriend's house in Crandon, Wisconsin. Six people were killed, including his ex-girlfriend; one was wounded. The shooter later committed suicide during an exchange of gunfire with police.

## Am-Pac Tire Pros (Commerce)

On October 8, 2007, at 7:30 a.m., Robert Becerra, twenty-nine, armed with a handgun, began shooting at customers and employees of Am-Pac Tire Pros in Simi Valley, California. One person was killed; two were wounded. The shooter committed suicide before police arrived.

## SuccessTech Academy (Education)

On October 10, 2007, at 1:02 p.m., Asa Halley Coon, fourteen, armed with two handguns, began shooting at SuccessTech Academy in Cleveland, Ohio. No one was killed; four were wounded. The shooter committed suicide before police arrived.

## Von Maur, Westroads Mall (Commerce)

On December 5, 2007, at 1:42 p.m., Robert Arthur Hawkins, nineteen, armed with a rifle, began shooting as he exited the elevator on the third floor of the Von Maur department store in the Westroads Mall in Omaha, Nebraska. Eight people were killed; four were wounded. The shooter committed suicide before police arrived.

## Youth with a Mission Training Center / New Life Church (House of Worship)

On December 9, 2007, at 12:29 a.m., Matthew John Murray, twenty-four, armed with a rifle, two handguns, and smoke bombs, entered the Youth with a Mission Training Center in Arvada, Colorado, and began shooting. Two people were killed; two were wounded. He then walked seven miles overnight to the New Life Church in Colorado Springs, Colorado, and began shooting again. Two additional people were killed there; three more were wounded. The shooter committed suicide after being shot by church security. A total of four people were killed; five were wounded.

# 2008
## Louisiana Technical College (Education)

On February 8, 2008, at 8:35 a.m., Latina Williams, twenty-three, armed with a handgun, began shooting in a second-floor classroom at Louisiana Technical College in Baton Rouge, Louisiana. She fired six rounds, then reloaded and committed suicide before police arrived. Two people were killed; no one was wounded.

## Cole Hall Auditorium, Northern Illinois University (Education)

On February 14, 2008, at 3:00 p.m., Steven Phillip Kazmierczak, twenty-seven, armed with a shotgun and three handguns, began shooting in the Cole Hall Auditorium at Northern Illinois University in DeKalb, Illinois. He had attended graduate school at the university. Five were killed; sixteen were wounded, including three who were injured as they fled. The shooter committed suicide before police arrived.

## Wendy's Fast Food Restaurant (Commerce)

On March 3, 2008, at 12:15 p.m., Alburn Edward Blake, sixty, armed with a handgun, began shooting in a Wendy's restaurant in West Palm Beach, Florida. One person was killed; four were wounded. The shooter committed suicide before police arrived.

## Atlantis Plastics Factory (Commerce)

On June 25, 2008, at 12:00 a.m., Wesley Neal Higdon, twenty-five, armed with a handgun, began firing at his coworkers in the Atlantis Plastics factory in Henderson, Kentucky. Prior to the incident, he was reprimanded by a supervisor for having an argument with a coworker and was escorted from the plant. He returned a brief time later and began shooting. Five people were killed; one was wounded. The shooter committed suicide before police arrived.

# 2009
## The Zone Nightclub (Commerce)

On January 24, 2009, at 10:37 p.m., Erik Salvador Ayala, twenty-four, armed with a handgun, began shooting at a crowd outside the Zone, an under-twenty-one nightclub in Portland, Oregon, and then shot himself before police arrived. He died in the hospital two days later. Two people were killed; seven were wounded.

## Coffee and Geneva Counties, Alabama (Open Space)

On March 10, 2009, at 4:00 p.m., Michael Kenneth McLendon, twenty-eight, armed with a rifle, killed five family members at various locations as he traveled through Coffee and Geneva Counties in southeast Alabama and continued shooting. A total of ten people were killed; one police officer was wounded. During an exchange of gunfire with police, the shooter committed suicide.

## American Civic Association Center (Commerce)

On April 3, 2009, at 10:31 a.m., Linh Phat Voong, aka Jiverly Wong, forty-one, armed with two handguns, began shooting in the American Civic Association Center in Binghamton, New York. He had previously taken classes at the center. The shooter blocked the back door of the building with his car and then entered through the front door. Thirteen people were killed; four were wounded. The shooter committed suicide before police arrived.

## Larose-Cut Off Middle School (Education)

On May 18, 2009, at 9:00 a.m., Justin Doucet, fifteen, armed with a handgun, fired once at a teacher at Larose-Cut Off Middle School in Cut Off, Louisiana, then went to the bathroom and shot himself. He died a week later. No one was killed or wounded.

## LA Fitness (Commerce)

On August 4, 2009, at 7:56 p.m., George Sodini, forty-eight, armed with three handguns, began shooting in an LA Fitness aerobics class at the Great Southern Shopping Center in Collier Township, Pennsylvania. He entered the gym, removed his guns from his gym bag, and began firing in the aerobics studio. Three people were killed; nine were wounded. The shooter committed suicide before police arrived.

## Legacy Metrolab in Tualatin, Oregon (Commerce)

On November 10, 2009, at 11:49 a.m., Robert Beiser, thirty-nine, armed with a handgun, a rifle, and a shotgun, began firing in the Legacy Metrolab in Tualatin, Oregon, his wife's place of employment. One week earlier, his wife had filed for divorce. His wife was killed; two were wounded. The shooter committed suicide before police arrived.

## 2010
## ABB Plant (Commerce)

On January 7, 2010, at 6:30 a.m., Timothy Hendron, fifty-one, armed with two handguns, a shotgun, and a rifle, began shooting at his coworkers in the parking lot at the ABB Plant in Saint Louis, Missouri, before moving into the building. He was a party in a pending lawsuit against his employer regarding the company's retirement plan. Three people were killed; five were wounded. The shooter committed suicide before police arrived.

## Farm King Store, Macomb, Illinois (Commerce)

On February 3, 2010, at 12:45 p.m., Jonathan Joseph Labbe, nineteen, armed with a rifle, began shooting inside a Farm King store in Macomb, Illinois. Eight people barricaded themselves in the office and remained hidden until police arrived. No one was killed or wounded. The shooter committed suicide after police arrived.

## Ohio State University, Maintenance Building (Education)

On March 9, 2010, at 3:30 a.m., Nathaniel Alvin Brown, fifty, armed with two handguns, began shooting in the maintenance building at Ohio State University in Columbus, Ohio. He had just been fired for allegedly lying on his job application. One person was killed; one was wounded. The shooter committed suicide before police arrived.

## Parkwest Medical Center, Knoxville, Tennessee (Health Care)

On April 19, 2010, at 4:30 p.m., Abdo Ibssa, thirty-eight, armed with a handgun, began shooting in the Parkwest Medical Center in Knoxville, Tennessee. He had been distressed over the outcome of his recent surgery and was trying to find his doctor, who he believed had implanted a microchip in him. When he was unable to find the doctor, he moved to the emergency room and began shooting. One person was killed; two were wounded. The shooter committed suicide before police arrived.

## Boulder Stove and Flooring (Commerce)

On May 17, 2010, at 11:05 a.m., Robert Phillip Montgomery, fifty-three, armed with a handgun, began shooting at the owners in the back office of Boulder Stove and Flooring in Boulder, Colorado. Two people were killed; no one was wounded. The shooter committed suicide before police arrived.

## Yoyito Café (Commerce)

On June 6, 2010, at 10:00 p.m., Gerardo Regalado, thirty-seven, armed with a handgun, began shooting in Yoyito Café in Hialeah, Florida, where his estranged wife was employed. Four people were killed, including his estranged wife; three were wounded. The shooter fled the scene and committed suicide several blocks away.

## Emcore Corporation (Commerce)

On July 12, 2010, at 9:30 a.m., Robert Reza, thirty-seven, armed with a handgun, began shooting in the Emcore Corporation building in Albuquerque, New Mexico, his girlfriend's place of employment. After confronting her, he began shooting throughout the building. Two people were killed; four were wounded, including his girlfriend. The shooter committed suicide once corporate security arrived.

## Hartford Beer Distribution Center (Commerce)

On August 3, 2010, at 7:00 a.m., Omar Sheriff Thornton, thirty-four, armed with two handguns, began shooting at his coworkers in the Hartford Beer Distribution Center in Manchester, Connecticut. He had been asked to quit for stealing beer from the warehouse. Eight people were killed; two were wounded. The shooter committed suicide after police arrived.

## AmeriCold Logistics (Commerce)
On September 22, 2010, at 9:54 p.m., Akouch Kashoual, twenty-six, armed with a handgun, began shooting at his coworkers in the break room of the AmeriCold Logistics plant in Crete, Nebraska. No one was killed; three were wounded. The shooter committed suicide before police arrived.

## Gainesville, Florida (Open Space)
On October 4, 2010, at 4:00 p.m., Clifford Louis Miller Jr., twenty-four, armed with a handgun, began shooting as he drove around Gainesville, Florida. One person, his father, was killed; five were wounded. The shooter committed suicide in a friend's driveway thirteen minutes after the shooting began.

## Panama City School Board Meeting (Education)
On December 14, 2010, at 2:14 p.m., Clay Allen Duke, fifty-six, armed with a handgun, began shooting during a school-board meeting in the Nelson Administrative Building in Panama City, Florida. The shooter's wife had previously been employed by the school district. After allowing several people to leave the room, the shooter fired in the direction of board members. No one was killed or wounded. The shooter committed suicide after being shot by the school district's armed security officer.

# 2011
## Millard South High School in Omaha, Nebraska (Education)
On January 5, 2011, at 12:44 p.m., Richard L. Butler Jr., seventeen, armed with a handgun, began shooting in Millard South High School

in Omaha, Nebraska. Earlier that day, the assistant principal had suspended the shooter for allegedly driving his car onto the football field. The assistant principal was killed; the principal was wounded. The shooter committed suicide after fleeing the site of the shooting.

## International House of Pancakes (Commerce)

On September 6, 2011, at 8:58 a.m., Eduardo Sencion, also known as Eduardo Perez-Gonzalez, thirty-two, armed with a rifle, began shooting in an International House of Pancakes in Carson City, Nevada. Three members of the US Air National Guard were killed, and two were wounded. In total, four people were killed; seven were wounded. The shooter committed suicide before police arrived.

## Southern California Edison Corporate Office Building (Commerce)

On December 16, 2011, at 1:30 p.m., Andre Turner, fifty-one, armed with a handgun, began shooting at his coworkers in a Southern California Edison corporate office building in Irwindale, California. Turner had just been told he would not receive a Christmas bonus and might be laid off. Two people were killed; two were wounded. The shooter committed suicide before police arrived.

## 2012
## McBride Lumber Company (Commerce)

On January 13, 2012, at 6:10 a.m., Ronald Dean Davis, fifty, armed with a shotgun, began shooting at his coworkers at McBride Lumber Company in Star, North Carolina. Three people were killed; one was wounded. The shooter shot himself at another location and later died in the hospital.

## Café Racer (Commerce)

On May 30, 2012, at 10:52 a.m., Ian Lee Stawicki, forty, armed with two handguns, began shooting inside Café Racer in Seattle, Washington, which he had been banned from entering because of previous incidents. He then fled to a parking lot, where he killed a woman to steal her car. Five people were killed; no one was wounded. The shooter committed suicide at another location.

## Sikh Temple of Wisconsin (House of Worship)

On August 5, 2012, at 10:25 a.m., Wade Michael Page, forty, armed with a handgun, began shooting outside the Sikh Temple of Wisconsin in Oak Creek, Wisconsin, and then moved inside and continued to shoot. The shooter exited the building and confronted the responding police officer, wounding him. He then fired on a second responding police officer, who returned fire and wounded the shooter. Six people were killed; four were wounded, including one police officer. The shooter committed suicide after being shot in the stomach by the second responding officer.

## Pathmark Supermarket, Old Bridge, New Jersey (Commerce)

On August 31, 2012, at 4:00 a.m., Terence Tyler, twenty-three, armed with a rifle and a handgun, began shooting at his coworkers in a Pathmark supermarket in Old Bridge, New Jersey. He returned after his shift dressed in military fatigues and carrying his weapons. He shot at a coworker outside the store, who ran inside and locked the door, warning other employees. The shooter gained entry to the store by shooting out the lock. Two people were killed; no one was wounded. The shooter committed suicide before police arrived.

## Accent Signage Systems (Commerce)

On September 27, 2012, at 4:35 p.m., Andrew John Engeldinger, thirty-six, armed with a handgun, began shooting in the Accent Signage Systems facility in Minneapolis, Minnesota. The shooter had just been fired from the company. Six people were killed; two were wounded. The shooter committed suicide before police arrived.

## Las Dominicanas M&M Hair Salon (Commerce)

On October 18, 2012, at 11:04 a.m., Bradford Ramon Baumet, thirty-six, armed with a handgun, began shooting in the Las Dominicanas M&M Hair Salon in Casselberry, Florida. The shooter had been served earlier that month with a domestic-violence court order involving his ex-girlfriend, who managed the salon. Three people were killed; his ex-girlfriend was wounded. The shooter committed suicide at another location.

## Azana Day Salon (Commerce)

On October 21, 2012, at 11:09 a.m., Radcliffe Franklin Haughton, forty-five, armed with a handgun, began shooting in the Azana Day Salon in Brookfield, Wisconsin, his estranged wife's place of employment. Three were killed, including his estranged wife; four were wounded. The shooter committed suicide before police arrived.

## Valley Protein (Commerce)

On November 6, 2012, at 8:15 a.m., Lawrence Jones, forty-two, armed with a handgun, began shooting at his coworkers in the Valley Protein processing plant in Fresno, California. The shooting took place midway through his shift. Two people were killed; two were wounded. The shooter committed suicide before police arrived.

## Clackamas Town Center Mall (Commerce)

On December 11, 2012, at 3:25 p.m., Jacob Tyler Roberts, twenty-two, armed with a rifle, began shooting at people waiting to see Santa Claus in the Clackamas Town Center Mall in Happy Valley, Oregon. Two people were killed; one was wounded. The shooter committed suicide before police arrived.

## Sandy Hook Elementary School and Residence (Education/Residence)

On December 14, 2012, at 9:30 a.m., Adam Lanza, twenty, armed with two handguns and a rifle, shot through the secured front door to enter Sandy Hook Elementary School in Newtown, Connecticut. He killed twenty students and six adults, and he wounded two adults inside the school. Prior to the shooting, the shooter killed his mother at their home. In total, twenty-seven people were killed; two were wounded. The shooter committed suicide after police arrived.

# 2013
## Osborn Maledon Law Firm (Commerce)

On January 30, 2013, at 10:45 a.m., Arthur Douglas Harmon III, seventy, armed with a handgun, began shooting during a mediation session at the Osborn Maledon law firm in Phoenix, Arizona. Two people were killed; one was wounded. The shooter later committed suicide at another location.

## Lake Butler, Florida (Open Space)

On August 24, 2013, at 9:20 a.m., Hubert Allen Jr., seventy-two, armed with a rifle and a shotgun, began shooting at his coworkers from Pritchett Trucking, Inc., as he drove around Lake Butler, Florida. He then returned home, where he committed suicide. Two people were killed; two were wounded.

## Sparks Middle School (Education)

On October 21, 2013, at 7:16 a.m., Jose Reyes, twelve, armed with a handgun, began shooting outside Sparks Middle School in Sparks, Nevada. A teacher was killed when he confronted the shooter; two people were wounded. The shooter committed suicide before police arrived.

## Arapahoe High School (Education)

On December 13, 2013, at 12:30 p.m., Karl Halverson Pierson, eighteen, armed with a shotgun, machete, and three Molotov cocktails, began shooting in the hallways of Arapahoe High School in Centennial, Colorado. As he moved through the school and into the library, he fired one additional round and lit a Molotov cocktail, throwing it into a bookcase and causing minor damage. One person was killed; no one was wounded. The shooter committed suicide as a school resource officer approached him.

## Renown Regional Medical Center (Health Care)

On December 17, 2013, at 2:00 p.m., Alan Oliver Frazier, fifty-one, armed with a shotgun and two handguns, began shooting in the Renown Regional Medical Center in Reno, Nevada. One person was killed; two were wounded. The shooter committed suicide at the scene after police arrived.

## 2014
## The Mall in Columbia (Commerce)

On January 25, 2014, at 11:15 a.m., Darion Marcus Aguilar, nineteen, armed with a shotgun and explosive devices, began shooting in the Mall in Columbia, Maryland, first in a retail store, then in the open mall. Two store employees were killed; five mall patrons were wounded. One person was shot in the ankle, and four others suffered other medical emergencies. The shooter committed suicide before law enforcement arrived.

## Fort Hood Army Base, Texas (Government)

On April 2, 2014, at 4:00 p.m., Ivan Antonio Lopez-Lopez, thirty-four, armed with a handgun, began shooting inside an administrative office on the Fort Hood Army Base in Texas. The active-duty soldier then moved (sometimes on foot, other times in a vehicle) from one location to another, firing inside and outside buildings. Three soldiers were killed; twelve were wounded. The shooter committed suicide after being confronted by a military law-enforcement officer.

## Federal Express (Commerce)

On April 29, 2014, at 5:50 a.m., Geddy Lee Kramer, nineteen, armed with a shotgun and explosive devices, began shooting at coworkers in a Federal Express sorting facility in Kennesaw, Georgia. He shot an unarmed security guard at the entrance control point and made his way into the facility, where he shot five more. No one was killed; six were wounded. The shooter committed suicide before law enforcement arrived.

## Residence and Construction Site in Jonesboro, Arkansas (Residence / Open Area)

On May 3, 2014, at 1:00 p.m., Porfirio Sayago-Hernandez, forty, armed with a handgun, began shooting at a friend's home in Jonesboro, Arkansas, killing two people and wounding four. The shooter then drove to a nearby construction site and killed one. A total of three people were killed; four were wounded. The shooter fled the scene and committed suicide at another location.

## Multiple Locations, Isla Vista, California (Open Space)

On May 23, 2014, at 9:27 p.m., Elliot Rodger, twenty-two, armed with a handgun and several knives, began shooting in the first of seventeen locations in Isla Vista, California. After stabbing three inside his apartment earlier that day, he began driving through town, shooting from his car. A total of six people were killed; fourteen were wounded. The shooter committed suicide after being wounded during an exchange of gunfire with law enforcement.

## Cici's Pizza and Walmart (Commerce)

On June 8, 2014, at 11:20 a.m., husband and wife Jerad Dwain Miller, thirty-one, and Amanda Renee Miller, twenty-two, each armed with a handgun (and one with a shotgun), began shooting at Cici's Pizza in Las Vegas, Nevada, killing two law-enforcement officers who were having lunch. The shooters took the officers' weapons and ammunition and fled to a nearby Walmart, where they killed an armed citizen who tried to intervene. Three were killed; no one was wounded. The male shooter was killed in an exchange of gunfire with law enforcement; the female shooter committed suicide during an exchange of gunfire with law enforcement.

## Reynolds High School (Education)

On June 10, 2014, at 8:05 a.m., Jared Michael Padgett, fifteen, armed with a handgun and a rifle, began shooting inside the boys' locker room at Reynolds High School in Portland, Oregon. One student was killed; one teacher was wounded. The shooter committed suicide after law enforcement arrived.

## United Parcel Service (Commerce)

On September 23, 2014, at 9:20 a.m., Kerry Joe Tesney, forty-five, armed with a handgun, began shooting in a UPS shipping facility in Birmingham, Alabama, from which he had recently been fired. Two supervisors were killed; no one was wounded. The shooter committed suicide before law enforcement arrived.

## Marysville-Pilchuck High School (Education)

On October 24, 2014, at 10:39 a.m., Jaylen Ray Fryberg, fifteen, armed with a handgun, began shooting in the cafeteria of Marysville-Pilchuck High School in Marysville, Washington. Four students were killed, including the shooter's cousin; three were wounded, including one who injured himself while fleeing the scene. The shooter, when confronted by a teacher, committed suicide before law enforcement arrived.

# 2015
## Melbourne Square Mall (Commerce)

On January 17, 2015, at 9:31 a.m., Jose Garcia-Rodriguez, fifty-seven, armed with three handguns, began shooting at his wife's workplace, Scotto Pizza, in Melbourne Square Mall in Melbourne, Florida. One person was killed; the shooter's wife was wounded. The shooter committed suicide before law enforcement arrived.

## Sioux Steel Pro-Tec (Commerce)

On February 12, 2015, at 2:00 p.m., Jeffrey Scott DeZeeuw, fifty-one, armed with a handgun, began shooting at coworkers at a steel mill in Lennox, South Dakota. One coworker was killed; two were wounded, including one who tried to intervene. The shooter fled the scene and committed suicide at another location.

## Walmart Supercenter (Commerce)

On May 26, 2015, at 1:00 a.m., Marcell Travon Willis, twenty-one, an active-duty US airman, armed with a handgun, began shooting at a Walmart Supercenter in Grand Forks, North Dakota. One store employee was killed; one store employee was wounded. The shooter committed suicide before law enforcement arrived.

## Grand 16 Theatre (Commerce)

On July 23, 2015, at 7:15 p.m., John Russell Houser, fifty-nine, armed with a handgun, began shooting moviegoers in the Grand 16 Theatre in Lafayette, Louisiana. Two people were killed; nine were wounded. The shooter committed suicide after law enforcement arrived.

## Syverud Law Office and Miller-Meier Limb and Brace, Inc. (Commerce)

On October 26, 2015, at 1:56 p.m., Robert Lee Mayes Jr., forty, armed with a handgun, began shooting at his estranged wife's workplace, Syverud Law Office, in Davenport, Iowa. The shooter then drove to Miller-Meier Limb and Brace, Inc., in nearby Bettendorf, where his estranged wife's father and an acquaintance were employed, and continued shooting. No one was killed; two were wounded. The shooter committed suicide after law enforcement arrived.

## 2016
## Knight Transportation Building (Commerce)

On May 4, 2016, at approximately 8:45 a.m., Marion Guy William, sixty-five, armed with a shotgun and a handgun, began shooting as he entered the Knight Transportation building in Harris County, Texas. The shooter, who had been fired from the company two weeks prior, killed a former coworker and then committed suicide. Two former coworkers were struck by shrapnel. One person was killed; two were wounded.

## The Plaza Live Theater (Commerce)

On June 10, 2016, at approximately 10:24 p.m., Kevin James Loibl, twenty-seven, armed with two handguns and a hunting knife, approached and fatally shot singer Christina Grimmie as she signed autographs during a meet-and-greet session after a concert at the Plaza Live Theater in Orlando, Florida. The suspect committed suicide after being tackled by the singer's brother. One person was killed; no one was wounded. Though only one person was killed, the assailant had multiple weapons, so it is believed he intended to continue killing.

# 2017
## Route 91 Harvest Music Festival (Open Space)

On October 1, 2017, millionaire businessman Stephen Paddock opened fire on the audience of the Route 91 Harvest Festival from the thirty-second floor of the Mandalay Bay Hotel and Casino in Las Vegas, Nevada, killing fifty-eight people and wounding over five hundred more. Paddock committed suicide when law enforcement determined which room he was in and was about to breach the door.

## First Baptist Church (House of Worship)

On Sunday, November 5, 2017, another horrifying mass killing occurred that took the lives of twenty-six people, including children, while they worshipped at the First Baptist Church in Sutherland Springs, Texas. The shooter, twenty-six-year-old Devin Kelley, a dishonorably discharged US Air Force service member with a history of violence against his family members and animals, entered the church and began randomly shooting. The shooter committed suicide after being shot and chased by a private citizen.

# Endnotes

1.  R. Osbaldiston, "'It Won't Happen to Me': The Optimism Bias," Eastern Kentucky University, March 2, 2016, http://psychonline. eku.edu/insidelook/%E2%80%9Cit-won%E2%80%99t-happen-me%E2%80%9D-optimism-bias.

2.  A. Griffin, "Clackamas Town Center Shooting: 22 Minutes of Chaos and Terror as a Gunman Meanders through the Mall," *Oregon Live*, December 15, 2012, http://www.oregonlive.com/clackamascounty/index.ssf/2012/12/clackamas_town_center_shooting_61.html.

3.  N. D. Weinstein, "Why It Won't Happen to Me: Perceptions of Risk Factors and Susceptibility," *Health Psychology* 3, no. 5 (1984): 431–57, https://www.ncbi.nlm.nih.gov/pubmed/6536498.

4.  "2000–2016 Active Shooter Incidents," FBI, accessed May 18, 2017, https://www.fbi.gov/file-repository/activeshooter_incidents_2001-2016.pdf/view.

5.  T. Bloom, "San Bernardino Elementary School Gunman 'Was Out for Blood,' Says Instructional Aide Who Witnessed Shooting," KTLA 5, April 13, 2017, http://ktla.com/2017/04/13/san-bernardino-elementary-school-gunman-was-out-for-blood-says-instructional-aide-who-witnessed-shooting/.

6.  F. Heinz, "Man Fires More than 100 Rounds at Police Headquarters," NBC 5, August 7, 2010, http://www.nbcdfw.com/news/local/Shots-Fired-Outside-McKinney-Police-Station-100886034.html.

7. C. Shoichet and G. Tuchman, "Chattanooga Shooting: 4 Marines Killed, a Dead Suspect and Questions of Motive," CNN, July 17, 2015, http://www.cnn.com/2015/07/16/us/tennessee-naval-reserve-shooting/index.html.

8. "A Study of Active Shooter Incidents in the United States between 2000 and 2013," FBI, accessed May 31, 2017, https://www.fbi.gov/file-repository/active-shooter-study-2000-2013-1.pdf/view.

9. "Massacre at Virginia Tech Leaves 32 Dead," History.com, accessed May 31, 2017, http://www.history.com/this-day-in-history/massacre-at-virginia-tech-leaves-32-dead.

10. "Army Major Kills 13 People in Fort Hood Shooting Spree," History.com, accessed May 31, 2017, http://www.history.com/this-day-in-history/army-major-kills-13-people-in-fort-hood-shooting-spree.

11. "Gunman Kills Students and Adults at Newtown, Connecticut, Elementary School," History.com, accessed May 31, 2017, http://www.history.com/this-day-in-history/gunman-kills-students-and-adults-at-newtown-connecticut-elementary-school.

12. A. Murgado, "Quicker Response to Active Shooters," *Police*, October 16, 2013, http://www.policemag.com/channel/patrol/articles/2013/10/quicker-response-to-active-shooters.aspx.

13. S. Chen, "San Diego Schools Could Cut 21 Officers Due to Budget Cuts," Fox 5, February 21, 2017, http://fox5sandiego.com/2017/02/21/san-diego-schools-could-cut-21-officers-due-to-budget-cuts/.

14. "A Study of Active Shooter Incidents in the United States Between 200 and 2013," FBI, September 16, 2013, https://www.fbi.gov/news/stories/fbi-releases-study-on-active-shooter-incidents.

15. "At Least 1 Student Shot at Texas High School, Female Shooter Dead," Fox News, September 8, 2016, http://www.foxnews.com/us/2016/09/08/shots-fired-at-texas-high-school-at-least-one-person-injured.html.

16. Associated Press, "Woman Kills 2 Students in Louisiana College Classroom, Takes Own Life," Fox News, February 8, 2008, http://www.foxnews.com/story/2008/02/08/woman-kills-2-students-in-louisiana-college-classroom-takes-own-life.html.

17. "Columbine High School Shootings," History.com, accessed May 31, 2017, http://www.history.com/topics/columbine-high-school-shootings.

18. "Active Shooter Incidents in the United States in 2014 and 2015," FBI, accessed December 9, 2017, https://www.fbi.gov/file-repository/activeshooterincidentsus_2014-2015.pdf/view.

19. M. Santia, "16-Year-Old Student Arrested following Quadruple Stabbing Outside Midtown School: NYPD," NBC New York, Accessed May 31, 2017, http://www.nbcnewyork.com/news/local/Four-Stabbed-Fight-Outside-NYC-School-Midtown-Teenagers-PS-35-NYPD-424265854.html.

20. R. Ellis, "Knife-Wielding Attackers Kill 29, Injure 130 at China Train Station," CNN, March 2, 2014, http://www.cnn.com/2014/03/01/world/asia/china-railway-attack/index.html.

21. Associated Press, "Man Stabs 22 Children in China," *New York Times*, December 14, 2012, http://www.nytimes.com/2012/12/15/world/asia/man-stabs-22-children-in-china.html.

22. K. Hall, "Knife-Wielding Attacker Kills Eight, Injures 15 at Japanese School," *Lubbock Avalanche Journal*, June 8, 2001, http://lubbockonline.com/stories/060801/upd_075-3395.shtml#.WTwkLIWcGUk.

23. J. Pearlman, "Australian Mother Who Killed Eight Children Suffered from Schizophrenia and Will Not Face Charges," *Telegraph*, May 4, 2017, http://www.telegraph.co.uk/news/2017/05/04/australian-mother-killed-eight-children-suffered-schizophrenia/.

24. M. McCrae, "Fifty Killed in a Knife Attack at a Chinese Colliery," Mining.com, October 1, 2015, http://www.mining.com/fifty-killed-in-a-knife-attack-at-a-chinese-colliery/.

25. "Nigeria: Riots Leave 500 Dead after Machete Attacks," *Telegraph*, March 8, 2010, http://www.telegraph.co.uk/news/worldnews/africaandindianocean/nigeria/7398142/Nigeria-riots-leave-500-dead-after-machete-attacks.html.

26. A. Myers, "Man Pleads Guilty to Mass Murder Involving Samurai Sword," *Honolulu Star Advertiser*, July 24, 2015, http://www.staradvertiser.com/2015/07/24/breaking-news/man-pleads-guilty-to-mass-murder-involving-samurai-sword/.

27. V. Dozier, "Bath Disaster: 89th Anniversary of Deadliest School Attack," *Detroit Free Press*, May 18, 2016, http://www.freep.com/story/news/local/michigan/2016/05/18/bath-disaster-89th-anniversary-deadliest-school-attack/84532530/.

28. E. McLaughlin, "Tourists Among 22 Killed in Apparent Attack on Bangkok Shrine," CNN, August 17, 2015, http://www.cnn.com/2015/08/17/asia/thailand-bangkok-bomb/.

29. "Fire Kills 87 People at the Happy Land Social Club in 1990," *Daily News*, March 17, 2015, http://www.nydailynews.com/new-york/nyc-crime/dozens-die-fire-illegal-bonx-social-club-1990-article-1.2152091.

30. "Nerve Gas Attack on Tokyo Subway," History.com, accessed May 31, 2017, http://www.history.com/this-day-in-history/nerve-gas-attack-on-tokyo-subway.

31. E. Emory, "Hot on the Trail of Cold 1911 Ax Murders," *Denver Post*, April 8, 2007, http://www.denverpost.com/2007/04/08/hot-on-the-trail-of-cold-1911-ax-murders/.

32. B. Berkowitz et al., "The Math of Mass Shootings," *Washington Post*, June 6, 2017, https://www.washingtonpost.com/graphics/national/mass-shootings-in-america/.

33. V. Kuo and P. Gast, "Rambling Gunman Dead after Opening Fire at Florida School Meeting," CNN, December 14, 2010, http://www.cnn.com/2010/CRIME/12/14/florida.meeting.shooting/index.html.

34. R. Sanchez, "Conn. Police Release Final Report on Newtown School Shooting," CNN, December 29, 2013, http://www.cnn.com/2013/12/27/justice/connecticut-newtown-shooting-report/.

35. "Mental Health Facts in America," National Alliance on Mental Health, accessed May 31, 2017, https://www.nami.org/Learn-More/Mental-Health-By-the-Numbers.

36. E. Friedman, "Va. Tech Shooter Seung-Hui Cho's Mental Health Records Released," ABC News, August 19, 2009, http://abcnews.go.com/US/seung-hui-chos-mental-health-records-released/story?id=8278195.

37. K. Yourish et al., "How Many People Have Been Killed in ISIS Attacks around the World," *New York Times*, July 16, 2016, https://www.nytimes.com/interactive/2016/03/25/world/map-isis-attacks-around-the-world.html.

38. "September 11, 2001: Background and Timeline of the Attacks," CNN, accessed May 31, 2017, http://www.cnn.com/2013/07/27/us/september-11-anniversary-fast-facts/index.html.

39. "Army Major Kills 13 People in Fort Hood Shooting Spree," History.com, accessed May 31, 2017, http://www.history.com/this-day-in-history/army-major-kills-13-people-in-fort-hood-shooting-spree.

40. J. Croft and T. Smith, "Dylann Roof Pleads Guilty to State Charges in Church Massacre," CNN, April 10, 2017, http://www.cnn.com/2017/04/10/us/dylann-roof-guilty-plea-state-trial/index.html.

41. J. Kandel and P. Healy, "20 Years Later: Bank-Robbing Duo Turned LA Neighborhood into a War Zone," NBC Los Angeles,

February 27, 2017, http://www.nbclosangeles.com/news/local/
Los-Angeles-Marks-20th-Anniversary-of-North-Hollywood-
Shootout-414756573.html.

42. "YouTube Video: Retribution," *New York Times*, May 24, 2014,
https://www.nytimes.com/video/us/100000002900707/youtube-
video-retribution.html?mcubz=0.

43. D. Thompson, "The Psychology of Elliot Rodger," PsychCentral.
com, accessed May 31, 2017, https://psychcentral.com/blog/
archives/2014/06/10/the-psychology-of-elliot-rodger/.

44. "Man Who Says He Was Omar Mateen's Gay Lover Speaks
Out," CBS, Accessed May 31, 2017, https://www.cbsnews.com/
news/orlando-shooting-man-who-says-he-was-omar-mateen-gay-
lover-speaks-out-univision/.

45. "Mindset," Dictionary.com, accessed May 31, 2017, http://www.
dictionary.com/browse/mindset.

46. G. de Becker, *The Gift of Fear: Survival Signals that Protect Us
from Violence*," January 20, 2010,

47. *The Bourne Identity*, directed by Doug Liman (2002: Hypnotic
Kennedy/Marshall, 2003), DVD.

48. A. Gallo, "How to Keep Your Team Focused and Productive during Uncertain Times," *Harvard Business Review*, March 8, 2017,
https://hbr.org/2017/03/how-to-keep-your-team-focused-and-
productive-during-uncertain-times.

49. "School Safety Tips," National Fire Protection Association, accessed May 31, 2017, http://www.nfpa.org/public-education/by-topic/property-type-and-vehicles/school-fires/school-safety-tips.

50. "Students Die in Chicago School Fire," History.com, accessed May 31, 2017, http://www.history.com/this-day-in-history/students-die-in-chicago-school-fire.

51. "School Building Fires (2009–2011)," Topical Fire Report Series, FEMA, accessed May 31, 2017, https://www.usfa.fema.gov/downloads/pdf/statistics/v14i14.pdf.

52. D. Grossman and L. Christensen, *On Combat, The Psychology and Physiology of Deadly Conflict in War and in Peace*, Warrior Science Publications, 3rd edition, October 1, 2008.

87746455R00093

Made in the USA
Columbia, SC
19 January 2018